OSCEs for
Obstetrics and Gynaecology

OSCEs for Obstetrics and Gynaecology

A. Pickersgill
MRCOG, MD
Consultant Obstetrician and Gynaecological Surgeon,
Stepping Hill Hospital, Stockport, Cheshire, UK

A. Meskhi
MRCOG
Staff Grade in Obstetrics and Gynaecology,
Wythenshawe Hospital, Manchester, UK

S. Paul
DFFP, MRCOG, MD
Specialist Registrar in Obstetrics and Gynaecology,
Furness General Hospital, Barrow-in-Furness, Cumbria, UK

BIOS

© BIOS Scientific Publishers Limited, 2001

First published 2001

A CIP catalogue record for this book is available from the British Library.

ISBN 1 85996 177 0

BIOS Scientific Publishers Ltd
9 Newtec Place, Magdalen Road, Oxford OX4 1RE, UK
Tel. +44 (0)1865 726286. Fax. +44 (0)1865 246823
World Wide Web home page: http://www.bios.co.uk/

Important Note from the Publisher
The information contained within this book was obtained by BIOS Scientific Publishers Ltd from sources believed by us to be reliable. However, while every effort has been made to ensure its accuracy, no responsibility for loss or injury whatsoever occasioned to any person acting or refraining from action as a result of information contained herein can be accepted by the authors or publishers.

The reader should remember that medicine is a constantly evolving science and while the authors and publishers have ensured that all dosages, applications and practices are based on current indications, there may be specific practices which differ between communities. You should always follow the guidelines laid down by the manufacturers of specific products and the relevant authorities in the country in which you are practising.

Production Editor: Andrea Bosher.
Typeset by Marksbury Multimedia Ltd, Midsomer Norton, Bath, UK
Printed by TJ International, Padstow, UK

CONTENTS

ABBREVIATIONS

AFP	alpha-fetoprotein
CISC	clean intermittent self-catheterization
CPD	cephalo-pelvic disproportion
CRH	corticotrophin releasing hormone
CRM	clinical risk management
CRP	c-reactive protein
CVP	central venous pressure
DI	detrusor instability
ECG	electrocardiogram
ECV	external cephalic version
FBS	fetal blood sampling
FDIU	fetal death in-utero
FISH	fluorescent *in situ* hybridization
FSH	follicle-stimulating hormone
GnRH	gonadotrophin-releasing hormone
GnRHa	gonadotrophin-releasing hormone analogue
GSI	genuine stress incontinence
hCG	human chorionic gonadotrophin
HELLP	haemolysis-elevated liver enzymes-low platelets
hMG	human menopausal gonadotrophins
HRT	hormone replacement therapy
ICP	integrated care pathway
IM	intramuscular
IUCD	intra-uterine contraceptive device
IUGR	intra-uterine growth restriction
MRC	Medical Research Council
NICU	neonatal intensive care unit
OHSS	ovarian hyper-stimulation syndrome
PMS	pre-menstrual syndrome
PPH	post partum haemorrhage
RCT	randomised controlled trial
RDS	respiratory distress syndrome
SCBU	special care baby unit
SHO	senior house officer
TED	thrombo-embolic deterrent

INTRODUCTION

The OSCE

Once you have passed the written part of the MRCOG examination you will be invited to attend the Objective Structured Clinical Examination (OSCE). This type of examination is designed to be fair to each candidate, in a reliable and valid way. It is designed to assess the width and depth of clinical skills. Although factual knowledge should have been proficiently tested in the written paper (by the MCQs and short essay questions), the OSCE will test it again. However, it is also designed to test history taking, examination skills, clinical understanding, problem-solving ability, investigation, diagnosis, treatment, counselling and communication skills. The examination lasts for 3 hours, with each candidate being given the same questions and oral assessment as everyone else. The OSCE circuit is divided into 'stations'. There are 12 stations in total, each one lasting for exactly 15 minutes. Two of the stations are 'rest' or preparatory stations. At these stations, the candidates may be given a piece of work to be discussed at the next 15-minute station. At all stations except the rest stations, there is a single examiner present, and at some stations a 'role-player' may also be present. These are often professional actors and actresses, briefed to play a particular role – perhaps an irate husband or a woman who is just about to be told her triple test is positive. Candidates will be assessed on their ability to take obstetric and gynaecological histories, counsel patients and demonstrate clinical skills. Remember to always be polite! At other stations candidates will be expected to critically appraise pieces of written work such as papers and information leaflets in discussion with examiners. At other stations candidates will be expected to discuss aspects of obstetrics, gynaecology and allied subjects in structured oral examinations.

The book

The book comprises a series of three OSCE circuits. Within each circuit there are 10 stations (A–J). Each of the stations may have different sections, which are represented numerically. The stations are designed to cover a wide range of topics and to try to develop the different skills that are required to be a competent doctor. It is not designed as a definitive text. Each question appears on a new page, and the remaining space on the page should be used to write down your answer. You should aim to complete each station in 15 minutes before moving on to the next one. The answers, where appropriate, have been referenced, but the references are suggested to be further reading. We have tried to use the principals of best practice and evidenced-based medicine to create the answers. Some of the answers represent my personal views and may not be found elsewhere; I take responsibility for that.

Of the three books that I have written, this has undoubtedly been the hardest. I have found it very difficult to try to mimic interactive stations, especially the counselling sessions, but trust I have achieved it. The words that I have used are ones that I normally use in my day-to-day practice and are there as a guide only. In the counselling questions the responses are written in what I consider to be a logical order. It may help if you can get someone else to read the responses and act as a role-player.

ACKNOWLEDGEMENTS

It has been a pleasure to work with Apollo and Sudipta again. They provided the suggestions for most of the questions and have been very supportive of my efforts to edit them. From inception to publication, this book has taken nearly 3 years. I am responsible for the delay because until now I was not entirely happy with it. I would like to apologise to Jonathan and the publishers for all the delays and to thank them for their patience.

I would like to thank Apollo and his wife Tini, and Sudipta for the enormous amount of work and time that they have put in to contribute to the book. Finally, I would like to thank Charlotte, my wife, for all her support and my daughter Jemima for being one of the reasons it has taken so long to finish this.

The sole reason for writing this book is to try to help people pass the examination, and hopefully it may also provide a way of improving your understanding and, most importantly, your care of your patients. I would be very grateful for any comments. Please e-mail me directly at Andypick@aol.com. Best of luck.

Andrew Pickersgill

NAMES OF MEDICAL SUBSTANCES

In accordance with directive 92/27/EEC, this book adheres to the following guidelines on naming of medicinal substances (rINN, Recommended International Non-proprietary Name; BAN, British Approved Name).

List 1 – Both names to appear

UK Name	rINN
[2]adrenaline	epinephrine
amethocaine	tetracaine
bendrofluazide	bendroflumethiazide
benzhexol	trihexyphenidyl
chlorpheniramine	chlorphenamine
dicyclomine	dicycloverine
dothiepin	dosulepin
eformoterole	formoterol
flurandrenolone	fludroxycortide
frusemide	furosemide
hydroxyurea	hydroxycarbamide
lignocaine	lidocaine
methotrimeprazine	levomepromazine
methylene blue	methylthioninium
mitozantrone	mitoxantrone
mustine	chlormethine
nicoumalone	acenocoumarol
[2]noradrenaline	norepinephrine
oxypentifylline	pentoxyifylline
procaine penicillin	procaine benzylpenicillin
salcatonin	calcitonin (salmon)
thymoxamine	moxisylyte
thyroxine sodium	levothyroxine sodium
trimeprazine	alimemazine
cephazolin	cefazolin
cephradine	cefradine
chloral betaine	cloral betaine
chlorbutol	chlorobutanol
chlormethiazole	clomethiazole
chlorathalidone	chlortalidone
cholecalciferol	colecalciferol
cholestyramine	colestyramine
clomiphene	clomifene
colistin sulphomethate sodium	colistimethate sodium
corticotrophin	corticotropin
cysteamine	mercaptamine
danthron	dantron
desoxymethasone	desoximetasone
dexamphetamine	dexamfetamine
dibromopropamidine	dibromopropamidine
dienoestrol	dienoestrol
dimethicone(s)	dimeticone
dimethyl sulphoxide	dimethyl sulfoxide
doxycycline hydrochloride (hemihydrate hemiethanolate)	doxycycline hyclate
ethacrynic acid	etacrynic acid
ethamsylate	etamsylate
ethinyloestradiol	ethinylestradiol
ethynodiol	etynodiol
flumethasone	flumetasone
flupenthixol	flupentixol
gestronol	gestonorone
guaiphenesin	guaifenesin
hexachlorophane	hexachlorophene
hexamine hippurate	methenamine hippurate
hydroxyprogesterone hexanoate	hydroxyprogesterone caproate
indomethacin	indometacin
lysuride	lisuride
methyl cysteine	mecysteine
methylphenobarbitone	methylphenobarbital
oestradiol	estradiol

List 2 – rINN to appear exclusively

Former BAN	rINN/new BAN
amoxycillin	amoxicillin
amphetamine	amfetamine
amylobarbitone	amobarbital
amylobarbitone sodium	amobarbital sodium
beclomethasone	beclometasone
benorylate	benorilate
busulphan	busulfan
butobarbitone	butobarbital
carticaine	articane
cephalexin	cefalexin
cephamandole nafate	cefamandole nafate

oestriol	estriol	sodium picosulphate	sodium picosulfate
oestrone	estrone	sorbitan monostearate	sorbitan stearate
oxethazaine	oxetacaine	stilboestrol	diethylstilbestrol
pentaerythritol tetranitrate	pentaerithrityl tetranitrate	sulphacetamide	sulfacetamide
		sulphadiazine	sulfadiazine
phenobarbitone	phenobarbital	sulphadimidine	sulfadimidine
pipothiazine	pipotiazine	sulphaguanadine	sulfaguanadine
polyhexanide	polihexanide	sulphamethoxazole	sulfamethoxazole
potassium clorazepate	dipotassium clorazepate	sulphasalazine	sulfasalazine
pramoxine	pramocaine	sulphathiazole	sulfathiazole
prothionamide	protionamide	sulphinpyrazone	sulfinpyrazone
quinalbarbitone	secobarbital	tetracosactrin	tetracosactide
riboflavine	riboflavin	thiabendazole	tiabendazole
sodium calciumedetate	sodium calcium edetate	thioguanine	tioguanine
sodium cromoglycate	sodium cromoglicate	thiopentone	thiopental
sodium ironedetate	sodium feredetate	urofollitrophin	urofollitropin

CIRCUIT 1

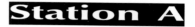

Question A1

You are covering the labour ward when a 30-year-old woman telephones for advice. She is currently 28 weeks pregnant, in her third pregnancy. She is worried because for the last 2 hours she has been getting some pains, roughly 10 minutes apart. The pain started 8 hours ago and has been increasing in frequency. She has two children aged 5 and 3 years. Both were delivered by lower segment caesarean section at term. The first caesarean section was performed for a breech presentation; the indication for the second was her previous section. The midwife advises her to come in for assessment.

On her arrival, how would you manage her, and if you thought that she was labouring, what would you do (explain this as though you were speaking to the patient)?

Your answer here ....

Question A2

Justify your choice of tocolytic. Can you tell me of any other drugs that you could use to prevent preterm labour progressing?

Your answer here ....

Question A3

Does delaying delivery improve neonatal outcome?

Your answer here ....

Question A4

Do you know of any methods currently available to predict preterm labour?

Your answer here ....

Question A5

Can preterm labour be prevented?

Your answer here ....

Question A6

Suppose you cannot prevent the progress of labour despite using ritodrine in this case. How would you manage her?

Your answer here ....

CIRCUIT 1

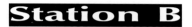

Question B1

How would you manage a unilateral, simple ovarian cyst, 5 cm in diameter, found by transvaginal ultrasonography in a 58-year-old postmenopausal woman referred by her GP?

Your answer here ....

Question B2

Do you know any other tumour markers that may be useful in this case?

Your answer here ....

Question B3

What is the role of transvaginal ultrasound in ovarian cancer screening?

Your answer here ....

Question B4

What ultrasound features suggest ovarian malignancy in postmenopausal women?

Your answer here ....

Question B5

This woman's CA125 comes back significantly raised. How would you now manage her case of suspected ovarian carcinoma?

Your answer here ....

Question B6

What are the reasons for taking peritoneal washings and removing the uterus and omentum?

Your answer here ....

Question B7

What are the reasons for performing debulking surgery even if the disease is incurable, and ideally what should be the optimal residue after debulking surgery?

Your answer here ....

CIRCUIT 1

Question C1

You are starting a family planning clinic at 10 a.m. on a Monday morning. The first client has already seen a nurse practitioner and has completed her history card. You read through this card before entering the room.

Pallantino Road Family Planning Clinic

Client number: 666
Name: *Emma Verymad*
Address: *2A, Fox Cottages, Nowhere-in-particular*
Age: *28*
Marital status: *Married*

GP Name: *Dr Katy Smallwood*
Address: *The Gifford House Surgery, Nowhere-in-particular*

Correspondence: ~~GP~~ / ~~Home~~ / None

L.M.P: *16 days ago*
Cycle: *3–4 / 28*
Current contraception: *Marvelon (day 10 of this packet)*
Previous contraception: *Barrier*

Previous genito-urinary diseases: *Genital warts 3 years ago*

Last cervical smear: *1 year ago – normal. Previous laser treatment*

Pregnancies: *TOP aged 23*

Illnesses or operations: *Occasional migraines. Depression*

Family history: *NAD*

Medications: *OCP, occasional paracetamol*

Smoker: *20/day*
Alcohol: *Socially*
Occupation: *Ultrasonographer*

Problem: *Forgot to take her pill last Friday morning, had unprotected sexual intercourse earlier that morning (02.00), whilst on a course from work (not with husband). Took two pills on Saturday morning. Worried may get pregnant, similar incident previously ended with unwanted pregnancy – terminated.*

What emergency contraception options are available, and which would suit her best?

Your answer here ....

Question C2

What would you have advised if the missed pill had been on either day 14 or day 20 of the packet?

Your answer here ....

Question C3

Having discussed the options with the woman she is still very anxious. Although the failure rate with the Yuzpe regime is higher at this late stage, she prefers to take that risk rather than having a coil inserted or trying the new levonelle pills. A friend has told her that she cannot have a coil because she has never had a baby, and is worried that her husband might notice the threads. She is also concerned that it will make her periods heavier and bring back her warts.

Counsel her in more detail about both of these methods, and try to reassure her.

Your answer here ....

Question C4

After your reassurance, Mrs Verymad decides that she would like a coil fitted. She also asks what you would advise for her future contraceptive needs.

Then explain to me exactly what you do when fitting a coil, and which particular coil you would use.

Your answer here ....

Question C5

During insertion of her coil, Mrs Verymad becomes sweaty, white and bradycardic. What would you do?

Your answer here ....

Question D1

A pharmaceutical company is launching a new drug called Detrusorstop for the treatment of urge incontinence. The representative comes to see you and your consultant at the end of a busy clinic. The new drug sounds very good, but you have not read any published articles about it. At the end of the meeting the representative leaves you with this information card. Read it and comment on it, including ways to improve it.

(Please note that this is a purely fictitious drug, company and journals.)

DETRUSORSTOP

Introducing the brand new once a week tablet to cure your patients with urge incontinence – Detrusorstop©. After millions of pounds of research and development Drug and Rep Pharmaceuticals are delighted to announce the arrival of Detrusorstop©. This highly efficacious, well tolerated, slow release anticholinergic has been specially formulated to increase compliance whilst at the same time increasing bladder capacity and decreasing that awful urge incontinence that plagues up to 40% of women.[1]

Tests and studies have proved that it is superior to placebo and other currently available pharmaceutical methods in the control of urge incontinence. Extensive published studies have proved beyond doubt that this is definitely the drug of choice in managing your patients.[2-3]

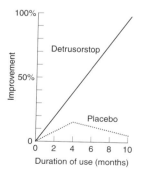

Detrusorstop can help to reduce your outpatient waiting times by reducing unnecessary follow up visits. As the graph clearly shows – the longer the duration of use the better the success rate, and therefore the better the compliance of your patients and the less visits they need.[4] In fact, Detrusorstop can be commenced following the diagnosis of detrusor instability at that first outpatient consultation.

When questioned 8 out of 10 women said they would prefer it.[5]

DON'T DELAY – ACT TODAY.
DETRUSORSTOP
TOGETHER WE CAN TAKE THE URGENCY OUT OF INCONTINENCE.

References:

1 Cardous O, Stress I, Cystos K. The debilitating effects of urge incontinence in a group of 30 pensioners. Manchester Incontinence Meeting 2000 (Abstract A10).

2 Dynamics URO and Cystogram Flo. Case report of the effect of the new slow release anticholinergic Detrusorstop on bladder control. Urogynaecological review 1999; **3**: 101-102.

3 Inconti NC. A pilot study comparing Detrusorstop to placebo for bladder capacity and voiding desire in post-menopausal women with urgency. Urogynaecological review 2000; **4**: 356-357.

4 Drug and Rep LTD. Detrusorstop verus placebo – continued decrease in urinary frequency with duration of use, in Rhesus monkeys following methotrexate instillation to mimic detrusor instability. Unpublished data.

5 Questionnaire survey regarding the success of currently available treatments for urge incontinence. Submitted for presentation.

Your answer here ....

Question D2

There has been a recent trend towards the development of evidence-based medicine. What do you understand by the term evidence-based medicine?

Your answer here ....

Question D3

Can you classify evidence into levels, if so how would you describe the levels?

The Royal College of Obstetricians and Gynaecologists grades its recommendations according to evidence. Do you know what these grades are?

Your answer here ....

Question D4

What do you understand by the term 'randomized controlled trial'? Can you give a current example? Why do these provide the best evidence? Do they have any disadvantages?

Your answer here ....

Question D5

What other ways do you know to minimize bias?

Your answer here ....

Question D6

What other factors can give misleading results?

Your answer here ....

Question D7

When evaluating a test, what is meant by the following terms:

True positive
True negative
False positive
False negative
Sensitivity
Specificity
Positive and negative predictive values
Relative risk
Likelihood (odds) ratio
Receiver operating characteristic curve
Bayes' theorem

Your answer here ....

Question D8

How do you assess the validity of a paper?

Your answer here ....

CIRCUIT 1

Question E1

A 25-year-old girl presents to the gynaecological ward late one night with an acute onset of abdominal pain and vomiting. She is otherwise well, expect for vague muscular pains and shoulder weakness. She had been at the pub with friends when the pain started. Her only medication was the oral contraceptive pill, which she has taken for the last 2 months. Her last period was 7 days ago. On examination she smells strongly of alcohol, is tachycardic and tender across her lower abdomen.

RESULTS:
Urinary Pregnancy test – negative

Urinalysis – no glucose or protein, but looks very dark on standing.

Ultrasound scan – normal sized anteverted uterus, endometrial thickness of 4 mm. Both ovaries seen and appear to be normal. No free fluid seen.

Haemoglobin	12.5 g/dl
White cell count	$13 \times 10^9/l$
Platelets	$155 \times 10^9/l$
Sodium	125 mmol/l
Potassium	5 mmol/l
Urea	6.5 mmol/l
Bilirubin	45 μmol/l
Aspartate transaminase	48 IU/l

What is your diagnosis? What test would you use to confirm this? What would be your management?

Your answer here ....

Your answer here (cont.) ....

Question E2 (i)

A couple with primary infertility (3 years duration) are being investigated. They are attending for their review appointment, to discuss their results.

25-year-old woman: Patent tubes on hysterosalpingography
Day 21 progesterone 45 nmol/l

29-year-old man: Semen analysis   Volume – 5 ml
No sperm seen

What is the likely cause of the infertility? What (if any) further tests would you recommend?

Your answer here ....

Question E2 (ii)

You repeat the man's semen analysis and check his hormonal profile. The results are:

Volume – 3 ml
Concentration – no sperm seen

Follicle stimulating hormone   23.2 IU/l
Luteinising hormone   19.4 IU/l

Prolactin   400 mU/l Q1

Testosterone   4.5 nmol/l

What is his diagnosis? What other investigations (if any) would you perform?

Your answer here ....

Question E3

The following are the results of a pre-operative screen on a 22-year-old woman admitted for a laparoscopy to investigate her pelvic pain and deep dyspareunia:

Haemoglobin	10.9 g/dl
Red blood cell count	$5 \times 10^{12}/l$
Packed cell volume	0.3 1
Mean corpuscular volume	62 fl
Mean corpuscular haemoglobin	22 g/dl
Mean corpuscular haemoglobin concentration	35 g/dl
Reticulocytes	2%
White cell count	$7 \times 10^9/l$
Platelets	$220 \times 10^9/l$
Serum iron	22 μmol/l
Total iron binding capacity	53 μmol/l

What is the likely diagnosis and how would you confirm this?

Your answer here ....

Question F1

Mrs Walker is a 29-year-old primigravida who is 10 weeks pregnant. She has come to Mr Smith's antenatal clinic (in a small district general hospital) for her booking visit. She has had her history taken by a midwife, who has also offered her the triple test (nuchal translucency is not available in your hospital). She feels she understands about the consequences of Down's syndrome and other chromosomal anomalies, but is worried and confused about the triple test, and wants to discuss it in detail with a doctor. You are the registrar (Dr Davies) in clinic; counsel her. Begin by checking her details and introducing yourself.

[This is a role-playing station, set as a simulated sequence of questions and answers in the antenatal clinic. Try and answer fully all Mrs Walker's questions and concerns. Begin as though you were meeting Mrs Walker for the first time. Her responses are in bold. Ask a friend to role play this station by reading out the bold type.]

Hello Mrs Walker, I am Dr Davies, Mr Smith's registrar. I understand from the midwife that you are concerned and confused about the triple test. I will try and answer your questions, and explain the test to you. Firstly, can I check your details please (name, address and date of birth)?

Hello Doctor. My name is Marie Walker, and I live at 34, Sandfield Road. My date of birth is August 10th. I want to know whether my baby is normal or not, but I am a bit confused about the triple test. Can you tell me more about the test please?

The triple test is a simple blood test. It is designed to give you an estimate of the risk of this baby being affected by Down's syndrome. **Q1** It does not say for definite whether or not this baby has Down's syndrome. It will identify about two thirds of babies with Down's syndrome. As I am sure that you are aware, the risk of having a baby with Down's syndrome increases with your age, but because more younger women than older women have babies, proportionally more Down's syndrome babies are born to young mothers. It is these affected babies that we hope to identify. Overall, the incidence of Down's syndrome is about 1 in 650 live births. The risk of you having a Down's syndrome baby at the age of 29 is approximately 1 in 1000.

The triple test measures the levels of three chemicals in your blood. These are the hormones oestriol (an oestrogen) and hCG (produced by the placenta, that makes your pregnancy test positive), and a protein called α-fetoprotein. The test is usually performed between 15 and 16 weeks of pregnancy. The timing is important because the chemical levels change as your pregnancy advances. The actual level of the chemicals when combined give an estimate of risk for Down's syndrome. When this is combined with how many weeks pregnant you are and the risk related to your age by the computer, it gives a final risk estimate. It does not say yes this pregnancy is OK or no it is not.

The main aim of the test is to divide pregnant women into two groups: those at high risk and those at low risk of a Down's syndrome baby. The cut-off point that we take is 1 in 250. So, if your risk were more than 1 in 250 (e.g. 1 in 150), you would fall into a high-risk group. If your risk were less than 1 in 250 (e.g. 1 in 700), you would be in a low-risk group.

What do you mean by high risk?

This means the probability of carrying a Down's syndrome baby is high enough to justify having an amniocentesis. As the risk of losing a baby following amniocentesis is about 1 in 200, the risk of carrying a Down's syndrome baby needs to be substantial for us to recommend an amniocentesis.

Does a low risk result mean I would have a normal baby?

No. It means that you still have 1 in something (less than 1 in 250) risk of carrying a Down's syndrome baby, but this risk does not justify having an amniocentesis, as the risk of losing a healthy baby would be greater than detecting a Down's syndrome baby. I have known women have a 1 in 2 risk from a triple test, but they have delivered normal babies; and I have known some women with very low risks (1 in 1500) give birth to babies affected by Down's syndrome.

So, I can't be sure whether the baby is normal or not unless I have the amniocentesis?

Yes that is correct.

What is an amniocentesis?

This is an investigation where we put a needle into the fluid around the baby. We then take some of this fluid and send it away to the microscope doctors **Q2**. They then grow the cells shed from the baby and are able to tell if the baby has normal chromosomes. Babies with Down's syndrome have an extra chromosome compared to normal.

Is it worth me having the triple test then?

I think that depends on your view of having a baby with Down's syndrome. If the baby was affected what would you do? Would you want to have a termination or would you carry on with the pregnancy? If you would continue with the pregnancy regardless, would you want to know if it was affected or not? A triple test would give you some idea about the risk of this pregnancy being affected, but the only definite answer would come from an amniocentesis. You need to decide what you would do if the triple test came back as positive, giving you a high risk of having a Down's syndrome baby. Unless you are decided about these issues, it may not be worthwhile having a triple test considering the anxiety associated with a positive test result.

Does the triple test help in detecting any other problem?

Yes. It is also a useful screening test for other chromosomal abnormalities (e.g. Edward's and Patau's syndrome etc.) and open neural tube defects (e.g. anencephaly, open spina bifida etc.).

Apart from the triple test and amniocentesis is there anything else I could have ?

Yes. You could have a chorionic villous biopsy. This is an invasive test, like an amniocentesis, but may carry a higher risk of miscarriage. Alternatively you could have an ultrasound scan to check the thickness of the skin on the back of the neck of the baby – this is called the Nuchal thickness. It also only gives a risk estimate of Down's syndrome. It is normally performed between 10 and 13 weeks of pregnancy, and is claimed to identify over three-quarters of affected babies.

Don't I have to have a scan before the triple test anyway – couldn't you measure the neck then?

You do need to have a booking scan to check that your baby is alright, and the age of the baby needs to be confirmed by scan before you have the triple test. Unfortunately, we do not perform the scans for nuchal thickness here. They are not routinely available in most hospitals, and further studies are being carried out to determine whether or not it is a reliable test for Down's syndrome.

Mrs Walker opts for a triple test and the report comes back as positive with a risk estimate of 1 in 40. She is now 17 weeks pregnant. A midwife has already telephoned her to inform her of the high risk, and she asks to see you again to counsel her.

Hello again Dr Davies. I've been told that my triple test has come back as positive, so what are we going to do now?

Yes Mrs Walker, I'm sorry to see you again under such unfortunate circumstances. Your triple test result is positive, with a risk estimate of 1 in 40. As I mentioned to you previously this puts you in the high-risk group. The only way now to rule out any chromosomal abnormalities in the baby is to perform an amniocentesis.

Suppose the amniocentesis shows an abnormal baby. What options do I have?

You would have two options, either to have a termination or to continue the pregnancy.

Do I have to have an amniocentesis?

No, not necessarily, unless you want to know whether the baby is affected or not. It is advisable to check the baby's normality, otherwise you may worry throughout the pregnancy. It is up to you whether you opt for amniocentesis or not.

When would I know whether the baby is normal or not?

It takes about 3 weeks for the laboratory to grow the cells.

Can't it be any quicker?

Yes, we could get the result in 3 days if we use a different and newer technique (FISH) for chromosomal analysis. This would look specifically for Down's syndrome and would not exclude other chromosomal abnormalities. It gives a preliminary result, which would later be confirmed by the result of cell culture.

Can't you check it just with the scan?

Some babies affected by Down's syndrome have abnormalities that may be picked up on scan – like for instance heart or intestinal defects. If we were to see one or more of these abnormalities it might be more suggestive of Down's syndrome, but still would not confirm the diagnosis. Similarly, Down's syndrome would not be excluded in absence of those abnormalities. So, really an ultrasound scan is not useful at this stage.

OK then, I would like to have the amniocentesis, but what are the risks involved?

The main risk following an amniocentesis is a miscarriage. This occurs on average once for every 200 amniocenteses performed. Other risks include harming the baby with the needle (to minimize this we scan you throughout), the development of an infection and the leakage of water from the baby's sac. If the water leak continues it may lead to a low volume of water around the baby. This can cause defects in the baby's feet (talipes) and hip (congenital dislocation of hip), which are correctable after birth, and lack of proper lung development (lung hypoplasia), which may cause problems with its breathing. There is also the chance that there may be some bleeding and if you have a Rhesus negative blood group we will need to give you an injection. Finally, there is a small (1–2%) chance of the cells not growing. If this happens we would need to repeat it.

Can you tell me what is involved in the procedure?

The procedure itself is normally straightforward. We begin by scanning your tummy to check that the baby is fine, to see where the afterbirth is and to find the space where most of the fluid is around the baby. We then clean your tummy to kill off any bugs and, whilst scanning at the same time we push a needle through your tummy into the womb. The needle will hurt the same as a needle placed in your arm when taking blood, it just seems strange that it is going into your tummy. Using a syringe we can then take a small amount of fluid from around the baby; removing this fluid does not harm the baby, because it is constantly producing more. We send the fluid off to the laboratory and wait for the result. The whole thing takes about 15 minutes. Once we have he results we would call you in and tell you in person. We would know whether or not the baby had Down's syndrome, and also its sex. Do you want to know the sex of the baby?

No, if it's all OK I want to enjoy the surprise at birth.

Fine. We would keep the report confidentially in the hospital notes.

Further reading

Chard T, Macintosh MCM (1994) Biochemical screening for Down's syndrome. In: Studd J (ed.), *Progress in Obstetrics and Gynaecology*, Vol. 11, pp. 39–52. Churchill Livingstone, Edinburgh.

Neilson JP (1995) Antenatal diagnosis of fetal abnormality and genetic disease. In: Whitfield CR (ed.), *Dewhurst's Textbook of Obstetrics and Gynaecology for Postgraduates*, 5th edn, pp. 121–139. Blackwell Science, Oxford.

Slade R *et al.* (1998) Prenatal diagnosis. *Key Topics in Obstetrics and Gynaecology*, 2nd edn, pp. 281–289.

Taylor AS, Braude PR (1994) Preimplantation diagnosis of genetic disease. In: Studd J (ed .), *Progress in Obstetrics and Gynaecology*, Vol. 11, pp. 3–22. Churchill Livingstone, Edinburgh.

Thornton JG (1993) Prenatal diagnosis. In: Studd J (ed.), *Progress in Obstetrics and Gynaecology*, Vol. 10, pp. 13–31. Churchill Livingstone, Edinburgh.

CIRCUIT 1

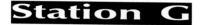

Question G1

A 25-year-old woman was referred to the gynaecological ward by her GP. The woman had recently undergone an IVF cycle, culminating with an embryo transfer 4 days ago. She had been infertile for 4 years prior to that. The cause of her infertility was felt to be a combination of her partner's low sperm count and anovulation. She was known to have polycystic ovaries, and was unsuccessfully treated with clomiphene citrate for 4 months. This was their first cycle of IVF. Following downregulation, human menopausal gonadotrophins (hMG) were used to induce multiple follicular growth. The oocyte recovery had harvested 12 eggs, of which seven had successfully fertilized. Three embryos had been replaced and the other four frozen. Following embryo transfer (and at the time of admission) she was on maintenance hCG injections.

On admission the woman was complaining of bloatedness, abdominal pain, thirst, vomiting and diarrhoea. She was in good general health. On examination, she was slim and she looked slightly pale. Her pulse was 82 beats per minute, blood pressure was 110/70 mmHg and temperature 36.8°C. Her abdomen was soft. There was some tenderness in the lower quadrants on palpation, but there were no signs of peritoneal irritation and no masses were palpable.

What is the likely cause of her symptoms and what is the form of presentation?

Your answer here ....

Question G2

What medications used in gynaecological practice are capable of causing this (separately or in combination)? What additional risk factors exist, especially with regard to her situation?

Your answer here ....

Question G3

What investigations would you perform and why – explain the pathophysiology?

Your answer here ....

Question G4

These are the results of your investigations.

Full blood count:

Haemoglobin	14.9 g/dl
Red blood cell count	5.3 x 10^{12}/l
Packed cell volume	0.51
Mean corpuscular volume	94 fl
Mean corpuscular haemoglobin	28 g/dl
Mean corpuscular haemoglobin concentration	30 g/dl
Reticulocytes	<1%
White cell count	11 x 10^9/l
Platelets	170 x 10^9/l

Urea and electrolytes:

Sodium	128 mmol/l
Potassium	5.1 mmol/l
Calcium	2.4 mmol/l
Chloride	97 mmol/l
Phosphate	1.2 mmol/l
Urea	10.2 mmol/l
Creatinine	140 μmol/l
Alkaline phosphatase	107 IU/l
γ-glutamyl transpeptidase	25 IU/l
Aspartate-amino transferase	34 IU/l
Alanine-amino transferase	28 IU/l
Bilirubin	7 μmol/l
Total protein	72 g/l
Albumin	33 g/l

Clotting screen:

Prothrombin time	12 seconds
Activated partial thromboplastin time	40 seconds

Chest X-ray: Normal

Abdomino-pelvic ultrasound scan:
The uterus is anteverted; the endometrial thickness is increased at 12 mm. Both ovaries are enlarged and contain multiple cysts. The right ovary measures 10 cm in diameter. The left ovary measures 9 cm in diameter. Free fluid was seen in the pelvis, but this does not appear to extend superiorly. The liver and kidneys appear normal. The gall bladder is normal.

Comment on the results and outline your initial management.

Your answer here ....

Question G5

Significant deterioration was observed over the subsequent 24 hours. Her abdominal girth increased by 3 cm, and her abdomen became tense. She developed progressive shortness of breath and a tachycardia. Her blood pressure declined to 100/60 mmHg. Despite your IV fluids she remained in negative fluid balance.

These are the results of your repeat biochemical and haematological investigations.

Full blood count:

Haemoglobin	16.9 g/dl
Red blood cell count	6.2×10^{12}/l
Packed cell volume	0.59
Mean corpuscular volume	95 fl
Mean corpuscular haemoglobin	27 g/dl
Mean corpuscular haemoglobin concentration	29 g/dl
Reticulocytes	$<1\%$
White cell count	16.2×10^9/l
Platelets	90×10^9/l

Urea and electrolytes:

Sodium	123 mmol/l
Potassium	5.5 mmol/l
Calcium	2.4 mmol/l
Chloride	97 mmol/l
Phosphate	1.2 mmol/l
Urea	12.2 mmol/l
Creatinine	148 μmol/l
Alkaline phosphatase	135 IU/l
γ-glutamyl transpeptidase	55 IU/l
Aspartate-amino transferase	40 IU/l
Alanine-amino transferase	39 IU/l
Bilirubin	7 μmol/l
Total protein	67 g/l
Albumin	28 g/l

Clotting screen:

Prothrombin time	16 seconds
Activated partial thromboplastin time	48 seconds

Comment on the results and her symptoms. What would be your criteria for a diagnosis of severe OHSS, and how would you treat it?

Your answer here ....

Your answer here (cont.) ....

Question G6

Do you know of any methods to prevent OHSS?

Your answer here ....

CIRCUIT 1

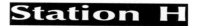

Question H1

You are called to the midwives' antenatal clinic to see a 28-year-old primigravid Nigerian solicitor attending her routine 36-week visit. The midwife has palpated her abdomen and thinks that this is a non-engaged breech presentation. What would you do?

Your answer here ....

Question H2

An ultrasound scan confirms a breech presentation with legs extended. The AC and HC lie on the 50th centile. The placenta is posterio-fundal and no pelvic masses are demonstrated. She knows that breeches are often delivered by caesarean section, but is keen to avoid this. She does not wish to be away from work for a long time or have unnecessary surgery.

Outline your discussion with her about the pros and cons of vaginal breech delivery.

Your answer here ....

Question H3

Following your discussion with her she asks if there is any way that the baby might turn by itself, or can you do anything to help?

Your answer here ....

Question H4

She opts for an ECV. Describe how you would perform one.

Your answer here ....

CIRCUIT 1

Question I1

A 56-year-old postmenopausal woman has come to the gynaecology clinic complaining of 'something coming down' in her vagina for 2 years. She also describes occasional pure stress incontinence for the last 6 months. She has three children, all of them were delivered vaginally. Her menopause was 5 years ago and she has never used any hormone replacement therapy. She has been treated for hypertension for the last 3 years; her blood pressure is now under control with frusemide. Apart from mild rheumatoid arthritis, she does not have any other significant medical or surgical history. There is a family history of breast carcinoma. General examination is unremarkable. On vaginal examination, you confirm that she has a moderate cystocele with first-degree uterine descent. No stress incontinence is demonstrable.

How would you manage her?

Your answer here ....

Question 12

What preoperative investigations would you perform before vaginal hysterectomy with repair in her case?

Your answer here ....

Question 13

Would you remove her ovaries and, if so, how?

Your answer here ....

Question 14

Suppose the lady comes back with a vaginal vault prolapse 2 years after a vaginal hysterectomy and anterior colporrhaphy. How would you manage her?

Your answer here ....

Question 15

What can you do at the time of hysterectomy to reduce the chance of vaginal vault prolapse?

Your answer here ....

Question J1

You have just begun your on-call shift at 5 p.m. on a Monday night. Prior to conducting a labour ward round, the bed manager informs you that there are no female beds in the hospital and you are not to accept any admissions that night.

At 18.30 you receive a call from a local GP who has just seen a 24-year-old caucasian woman in his surgery. She is complaining of lower abdominal pain and small, but recurrent vaginal bleeds over the last few days. Previously, she had one normal delivery and two early miscarriages. She had been using the combined oral contraceptive pill until 3 months ago. She was suffering from breakthrough bleeding, migraines and bloating; consequently she now has a copper coil *in situ*. Since the coil has been inserted she has continued to have irregular vaginal bleeding. She thinks her last menstrual period was 3 weeks ago. She is single, unemployed and lives in a council flat with her 2-year-old daughter. She smokes 25–30 cigarettes per day. She is otherwise in good general health.

On examination she looks well and her observations are stable. Her abdomen is soft, non-tender, with no signs of peritoneal irritation. On vaginal examination the uterus is slightly bulky, anteverted and mobile. There is some tenderness on cervical motion and some tenderness in the right adnexae. There are no pelvic masses palpable.

The GP has done a urinary pregnancy test that is positive. He is obviously concerned about the viability and nature of the pregnancy and wishes to send her in to you. She will need to bring her daughter with her because she cannot arrange alternative child care.

In view of the instructions of the bed manager, what would you do, bearing in mind that you have 24-hour access to a transvaginal scan and you are competent in scanning early pregnancies for viability?

Your answer here ....

Your answer here (cont.) ....

Question J2

Despite the fact that you are not allowed to admit anyone, you see no reason not to arrange for her to come in for a scan. A high-resolution transvaginal ultrasound scan shows a sac in the uterus under 0.2 ml in volume, but no fetal pole is seen. Both ovaries were seen and appeared normal and no adnexal pathology was identified. No free fluid was noted in her pouch of Douglas. The coil is noted to be present, and posterior to the sac.

What ultrasonic features help to distinguish between an intrauterine pregnancy and a tubal pregnancy at this gestational stage?

How would you counsel this woman, and subsequently manage her?

Your answer here ....

Question J3

What are the disadvantages of diagnostic laparoscopy at this stage?

Your answer here ....

Question J4

At review 2 days later, the woman remains generally well, although her abdominal pain has got slightly worse and is now localized to the left iliac fossa. There has been no further vaginal bleeding noted. The results of the two quantitative beta hCG measurements are (at 48-hour intervals) respectively 856 IU/l and 1296 IU/l. A repeat ultrasound scan is unhelpful, with no intrauterine changes noted. A small amount of free fluid is noted posterior to the uterus.

In view of the results and her increasing pain, a laparoscopy was performed. This revealed a normal uterus and right adnexae. Her left ovary was normal, but the left tube was enlarged to 2 cm diameter, 3 cm from the cornual end. It was a cherry colour and intact. There were 20–30 ml of pink fluid in the pouch of Douglas.

What management options are now available?

Your answer here ....

Question J5

A partial salpingectomy was performed and following this she made a good recovery. Histology confirmed a tubal pregnancy.

How would you counsel her with regard to her future fertility and contraception?

Your answer here ....

CIRCUIT 1

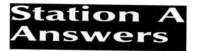

Answer A1

On her arrival, I would introduce myself to her (and her partner if present). I would then take a thorough history, paying particular attention to risk factors associated with pre-term labour. I would be interested in the site and nature of the pain, the presence of any uterine contractions (and any pain between them), vaginal loss (bleeding or discharge), urinary and bowel symptoms and fetal movements. I would also look through her antenatal notes to help me to obtain adequate knowledge about this pregnancy, particularly to confirm the gestational age, the number and the normality of the fetus, and the site of the placenta (from the anomaly scan). I would also check for the presence of any complicating factors in this pregnancy.

After taking her history, I would perform general, abdominal and vaginal examinations. General examination would include assessment of her temperature, colour, pulse, and blood pressure. I would examine her abdomen to assess the uterus (height of the fundus in cm, contractions, consistency between contractions, and tenderness, especially over the scar), and its contents (the lie and presentation of the fetus, liquor volume, fetal movements and heart rate). I would perform a speculum examination to look for bleeding, discharge or drainage of liquor and any cervical change. I would take a high vaginal swab for culture and sensitivity and an intracervical swab for chlamydia. If there is no evidence of a placenta praevia I would perform a vaginal examination to assess the cervix.

If obvious signs of labour were present (such as dilatation and effacement of the cervix), and I had excluded other causes of abdominal pain (e.g. scar dehiscence, placental abruption, urinary tract infection), I would explain to the woman that she appeared to be in 'pre-term' labour. Then I would begin to counsel her with regard to the risks (increased perinatal morbidity and mortality) associated with giving birth to a 28-week-old baby.

I would explain that the main problem facing a child born at this gestational age would be that its lungs are not fully mature. Thus, it would have a more than one in two chance (>50%) of developing respiratory distress syndrome (RDS), which is a significant cause of death and severe morbidity in pre-term infants. After delivery, her baby would need admission to the neonatal intensive care unit (NICU)/special care baby unit (SCBU), where it would probably require ventilation. To help her baby's lungs mature and to reduce the risk of RDS (by 40–60%), we could give her steroid injections. The steroids would cross the placenta and help to mature the baby's lungs. Steroids have most benefit after 24 hours, so we should try to delay delivery for at least 24 hours to allow the steroids to act, and transfer her to a unit with NICU (if not provided in this hospital). I would also explain that steroids reduce the chances of a brain (intra-ventricular) haemorrhage from occurring within an hour of administration, and seem to reduce the risks of necrotizing enterocolitis – a potentially fatal condition of the bowel. If she does not deliver then giving her steroids would not cause her baby harm. I would also reassure her that there are few risks to herself. If she were in agreement I would prescribe a dose of betamethasone 12 mg to be given intramuscularly (IM) immediately, and to be repeated after 24 hours. (An alternative is 4 doses of dexamethasone 6 mg IM given 12 hours apart.)

I would then explain that we needed to give her ritodrine – a drug used to stop uterine contractions. This is given intravenously and requires a drip in her arm (intravenous line). Its main side effect is to increase her heart rate, which may cause her to feel palpitations. Before commencing, I would obviously exclude any contraindications (such as heart disease, thyrotoxicosis etc.).

If there were evidence of maternal infection I would commence her on antibiotics. If there were no evidence of maternal infection I would not (ORACLE trial)

If there was no obvious sign of labour and she continued to have regular uterine contractions I would re-assess the cervical condition in 2 hours and consider ritodrine if there had been a significant change. I would still give her steroids.

I would inform SCBU of her admission and assessment, and to ensure that they are happy to take the baby in case she delivers. If they are full or if the facility to look after a 28-week-old baby is lacking, I would arrange for an *in utero* transfer to an appropriate neonatal unit. I would keep the paediatricians informed of her progress. If they were not busy I would ask either one of them or a member of their team to come and talk to the woman in more detail about the problems of prematurity and the long-term outlook if her baby is born.

Answer A2

Betamimetics are used more extensively than any other drug in this country for inhibiting labour. Ritodrine has been studied more fully than the other drugs in this class in controlled trials, and it has proved to be effective in delaying delivery beyond 48 hours in preterm labour (although they do not decrease perinatal mortality or serious morbidity).

NB. You could have suggested using prostaglandin synthesis inhibitors like indomethacin, which have been shown to be more effective in inhibiting myometrial contractility than betamimetic drugs. They may also reduce the risks of preterm birth and low birthweight, and there is a trend towards them reducing the incidence of respiratory distress syndrome and perinatal death. Alternatively, a calcium channel blocker such as nifedipine could be used, which has also been shown to be effective in a randomized multi-centre trial.

Many drugs have been tested as tocolytics, but few are effective. Some of them have been used in clinical practice and some are still at the research stage:

- **Other betamimetics,** such as salbutamol and terbutaline are effective, but have never been popular in the UK.

- **Prostaglandin synthetase inhibitors** (non-steroidal anti-inflammatory agents) such as indomethacin are effective, but are associated with renal dysfunction, premature closure of the ductus arteriosus, intracerebral haemorrhage and necrotizing enterocolitis (possibly secondary to chronic lung disease) in the neonate.

- **Calcium channel blockers,** such as nifedipine, are also effective. A recent metanalysis has shown that they appear to be more effective than beta-agonists for tocolysis and have a better side effect profile. However, they are associated with decreased uterine blood flow and oxygen saturation in the fetus leading to fetal acidosis. They also affect placental vasculature and need further evaluation.

- **Magnesium sulfate** is comparable to ritodrine, but has never been popular in the UK because of the need for cautious use. Placebo controlled trials have not confirmed its usefulness in reducing the frequency of adverse outcomes.

- The **oxytocin antagonist** (Atosiban) has been shown to reduce the frequency of uterine contractions but not the progress of preterm labour and needs further evaluation.

- **Nitric oxide donors,** such as sodium nitroprusside, seem to be promising, but the results of trials are awaited to confirm this.

- **Potassium channel openers** may show some prospect for the future.

The use of progestogen, ethanol or Diazoxide is no longer justified.

Answer A3

No. Delaying delivery alone does not seem to improve the neonatal outcome, but it provides time for the steroids to act. Steroids reduce the incidence of respiratory distress syndrome, intraventricular haemorrhage and death in the neonate. They also enhance the efficacy of neonatal surfactant therapy.

Answer A4

Several methods have been tested, but most of them are not useful, except perhaps fetal fibronectin found in cervico-vaginal secretions. A positive test at 22–24 weeks predicted 60% of spontaneous preterm births less than 28 weeks. (Overall, fetal fibronectin has 70–80% sensitivity, 70–80% specificity, 30% positive predictive value and 95% negative predictive value. False positive result may occur due to contamination with amniotic fluid or blood.)

Risk scoring has been devised, but it is not very useful (sensitivities and positive predictive values in the range of 20–30%). It incorporates factors such as race, socio-economic status, previous preterm birth, multiple pregnancy, extremes of reproductive life, smoking, alcohol intake, cocaine use, assisted conception, manual work, working long hours, general medical and obstetrical disorders

Cervical assessment by transvaginal scan or bimanual examination has been assessed, but the cut-off point for cervical length is ill defined. Although these measurements may be useful in singleton pregnancies, in twins they are less useful (in an unselected population the positive predictive value for preterm labour was only 26%).

Uterine activity monitoring has been shown to increase birth weight and to improve neonatal morbidity, and needs further studies.

Biochemical markers such as increased salivary estriol, estriol/progesterone ratio, serum collagenase, plasma CRH and serum relaxin need further evaluation.

Infections and mediators of inflammation such as bacterial vaginosis, *Trichomonas vaginalis*, ureaplasma, *B. fragilis*, leukocytes, leukocyte esterase, cytokines, glucose concentration and zinc need further evaluation.

Increased CRP, Mycoplasma and lipocortin-1 have not been shown to have significant predictive value.

Answer A5

No. At present there are no methods available in clinical practice to effectively prevent preterm labour.

- **Magnesium** has been shown to reduce the incidence of preterm labour, but not perinatal mortality.

- **Calcium** may reduce preterm birth, but the role of routine supplementation is not clear.

- **17 alpha-hydroxyprogesterone caproate** has been shown to reduce the incidence of preterm labour and preterm birth, but needs further evaluation.

- There is no evidence that **social support** and **betamimetic drugs** are effective.

- **Bed rest** has no value except in triplets and multiple pregnancies of greater order; paradoxically, it has been shown to increase the incidence of preterm labour in twins.

- **Cervical cerclage** can prevent one preterm labour out of 25 procedures (MRC trial), so it is practically not useful.

Answer A6

I would explain to the woman there is a risk of scar rupture (1.2%) if vaginal delivery is contemplated, against the risks of a third caesarean section. In view of her history of two previous caesarean sections, I would suggest delivery again by caesarean, preferably under spinal anaesthesia. I would also explain the possibility of a classical section in case the lower segment was not well formed. I would discuss the proposed management with the on-call consultant obstetrician (his/her presence may be required if the registrar were less experienced). I would also contact the on-call paediatrician to confirm that he/she is happy to receive the baby.

Further reading

Enkin MW, Keirse MJNC, Renfrew MJ, Neilson JP (1995) Preterm labour. In: *A Guide to Effective Care in Pregnancy and Childbirth*, 2nd edn, pp. 161–173. Oxford University Press, Oxford.

Kenyon SL, Taylor DL, Tarnow-Mordi W (2001) Broad-spectrum antibiotics for pre-term, prelabour rupture of the fetal membranes: the ORACLE I randomised trial. ORACLE Collaborative Group. *Lancet* **357**: 979–988.

Kenyon SL, Taylor DL, Tarrow-Mordi W (2001) Broad-spectrum antibiotics for spontaneous preterm labour: the ORACLE II randomised trial. ORACLE Collaborative Group. *Lancet* **357**: 989–994.

Lamont RF, Fisk N (1993) The role of infection in the pathogenesis of preterm labour. In: Studd J (ed.), *Progress in Obstetrics and Gynaecology,* Vol. 10, pp. 135–158. Churchill Livingstone, Edinburgh.

Meehan FP, Rafla NM, Bolaji **Q4** (1993) Delivery following previous caesarean section. In: Studd J (ed.), *Progress in Obstetrics and Gynaecology,* Vol. 10, pp. 213–228. Churchill Livingstone, Edinburgh.

Morrison JJ (1996) Prediction and prevention of preterm labour. In: Studd J (ed.), *Progress in Obstetrics and Gynaecology,* Vol. 12, pp. 67–85. Churchill Livingstone, Edinburgh.

Ritchie JWK (1995) Obstetric operations and procedures. In: Whitfield CR (ed.), *Dewhurst's Textbook of Obstetrics and Gynaecology for Postgraduates*, 5th edn, pp. 388–400. Blackwell Science, Oxford.

Royal College of Obstetricians and Gynaecologists (1996) Antenatal corticosteroids to prevent respiratory distress syndrome. RCOG Guideline, No. 7.

Royal College of Obstetricians and Gynaecologists (1997) Beta-agonists for the care of women in preterm labour. RCOG Guideline, No. Ia.

Slade *et al.* (1998) Premature labour. In: *Key Topics in Obstetrics and Gynaecology*, pp. 276–280. BIOS Scientific Publishers Ltd, Oxford.

Tsatsaris V, Papatsonis D, Goffinet F, Dekker G, Carbonne B (2001) Tocolysis with nifedipine or beta-adrenergic agonists: a meta-analysis. *Obstetrics and Gynaecology* **97**: 840–847.

CIRCUIT 1

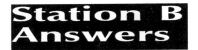

Answer B1

Having read the scan report, I would wish to take a full history and examine the woman myself. In the history I would try and ascertain if she had any symptoms related to malignancy – such as decreased appetite and weight loss, or a family history of breast, ovarian or colonic carcinoma. I would also look for risk factors for ovarian cancer, such as nulliparity. My examination would include a breast examination and a vaginal examination to see if the cyst was still present, and if so its consistency, mobility etc.

Initially I would explain that although the scan has suggested that this cyst is ovarian in origin it could be wrong. The cyst could be something else, like a pedunculated fibroid, a swollen tube (hydrosalpinx), a parafimbrial cyst or a peritoneal cyst. I would also explain to the woman that the presence of an ovarian cyst is not common after the menopause and further investigations are necessary to try and exclude any suggestion of malignancy. I would try to reassure her that as the cyst appears to be unilateral and simple, there is nothing to suggest malignancy on scan. However, I would also point out that there is no test currently available to adequately diagnose ovarian cancer.

If she wished we could treat her conservatively and monitor the cyst both biochemically and with further scans. In the presence of a normal serum CA125 measurement, about 50% of simple cysts regress after 6 months. If regression did not occur, I would then repeat the transvaginal scans every 6 months for three years, as 99% of simple cysts regress by that time. If the cyst does not regress or becomes larger at 6 months, I would repeat a serum CA125 measurement to help predict the outcome.

If she was anxious and unhappy to be monitored, or had high risk factors I would offer her a laparoscopy.

Answer B2

Serum CA19-9 and carcinoembryonic antigen (CEA) measurements at the initial diagnosis are useful to predict future regression of the cyst.

Answer B3

Transvaginal ultrasonography is simple, safe and relatively cheap to perform, hence it is a popular screening method at present. It produces images of greater resolution and better quality than the transabdominal approach. This is mainly because the transducer is closer to the organs and there is not the interference generated by fat and muscle, so ultrasound of higher frequencies can be used. A full bladder is not required and many women prefer this.

The disadvantages are that it is more invasive than transabdominal scans, with limited access and poor patient acceptability if there is postmenopausal vaginal atrophy. The penetration is limited to 10 cm due to the high frequencies used. Thus, ovaries situated very high or lateral in the pelvis, or that are grossly enlarged may not be seen.

Although it is very sensitive, it has poor specificity. So, it is not recommended for use alone as a screening method (it has a 1.2% positive predictive value for the detection of asymptomatic early ovarian cancer). The positive predictive value can be improved by combining colour Doppler study and measuring serum tumour markers along with the transvaginal scan.

Answer B4

Features suggestive of ovarian malignancy include

- a large mass where the ovarian volume is above the 99.5th percentile, more than twice the overall mean, or more than twice that of its pair;

- a cyst/mass with an irregular outline, showing surface papillary growths;

- a cyst/mass that appears to be either hypo- or hyperechogenic;

- if it is semi-solid/semi-cystic with thick septa it is unlikely to be simple;

- bilateral cysts (these are highly suggestive of malignancy);

- metastatic disease may be found with ascites, hydronephrosis (rarely), an omental 'cake' and matted bowel loops;

- the endometrium may be thickened with a co-existing endometrial tumour.

Answer B5

I would explain the provisional diagnosis and the treatment options to the patient. The optimal treatment is surgery, with removal of the ovary with the tumour, the other ovary, the uterus, both fallopian tubes and the omentum. I would explain the operative procedure and its complications to her and arrange an urgent admission (within 6 weeks).

I would then check her full blood count and serum urea, electrolytes and creatinine levels. I would also ask for liver function tests to be performed. I would request two units of blood. In view of her age I would arrange a chest X-ray and electrocardiogram (ECG) and other preoperative investigations as necessary. I would ask for a preoperative assessment to ascertain her anaesthetic fitness. I would gain her consent and I would wish her to have pre-operative bowel preparation in case of bowel involvement at laparotomy.

The operation itself is a staging laparotomy through a vertical lower abdominal incision, which can be extended above the level of the umbilicus if necessary. The aims of the primary surgery are to confirm the diagnosis, to stage the disease and to remove the malignant tissue as much as possible. If ascitic fluid is present, it should be sent for cytological examination. In its absence, 100 ml of normal saline should be instilled into the paracolic gutters and the pouch of Douglas and subsequently withdrawn for cytological examination. The tumour, other ovary, uterus, both tubes, peritoneal surfaces, large and small bowels, liver, undersurface of the diaphragm, para-aortic lymph nodes and the omentum should be examined to confirm and to accurately stage the disease. The usual operation consists of total abdominal hysterectomy, bilateral salpingo-oophorectomy with infracolic omentectomy and biopsy of any suspicious para-aortic lymph nodes. In case of widespread disease, removal of as much malignant tissue as possible should be undertaken (debulking).

Answer B6

Peritoneal washings are positive in 10–50% of apparently early (stage I and II) disease.

The rationale for removing the uterus is that it is a common site for lymphatic metastases, there is an increased chance of serosal and endometrial implants and an increased risk of developing endometrial cancer in future. It is also part of the debulking procedure.

The rationale for removing the omentum is partly for staging, removal of potential site of metastasis and future recurrence, and to reduce the chance of ascites due to omental caking.

Answer B7

Even if the disease is incurable, debulking surgery is performed to relieve symptoms such as reducing the distress from the pressure effect, and to enhance the effects of chemotherapy. It will increase the sensitivity of the tumour to subsequent chemotherapy as large tumours have poor oxygenation, lower growth fraction and relative insensitivity to chemotherapy. It will also improve the host immune response. For optimal response the remaining tumour should be less than 2 cm in diameter.

Further reading

Jacobs I (1996) The impact of molecular genetics in gynaecological cancer. In: Studd J (ed.), *Progress in Obstetrics and Gynaecology*, Vol. 12, pp. 421–448. Churchill Livingstone, Edinburgh.

Peel KR (1995) Benign and malignant tumours of the ovary. In: Whitfield CR (ed.), *Dewhurst's Textbook of Obstetrics and Gynaecology for Postgraduates*, 5th edn, pp. 759–779. Blackwell Scientific Publishers, Oxford.

Prys Davies A, Oram D (1991) Screening for ovarian cancer. In: Studd J (ed.), *Progress in Obstetrics and Gynaecology*, Vol. 9, pp. 349–373. Churchill Livingstone, Edinburgh.

Sasaki H *et al.* (1999) Follow up of women with simple ovarian cysts detected by transvaginal sonography in the Tokyo metropolitan area. *Br. J. Obstet. Gynaecol.* **106**: 415–420.

Slade R *et al.* (1998) Ovarian tumours. *Key Topics in Obstetrics and Gynaecology* 2nd edn. BIOS Scientific Publishers Ltd, Oxford, pp. 87-92.

CIRCUIT 1

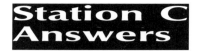

Answer C1

She had unprotected intercourse at 02.00 last Thursday night/Friday morning – this was 80 hours ago. Today she is on day 10 of this packet of Marvelon. At the time of intercourse she would have taken 6 days of her pills. It is generally accepted that 7 days of pill intake are required to render ovaries quiescent, therefore there is a slight danger that she might ovulate this cycle and become pregnant. Should she have been a further day into her packet she would not require any further treatment.

The commonest post-coital method 'The Yuzpe regime' (100 µg of ethinylestradiol and 500 µg of levonorgestrel) should be commenced within 72 hours of the act of unprotected intercourse. After 72 hours its success rate diminishes, but it is not contra-indicated. The more recently licensed Levonelle-2 (levonorgestrel 0.75 mg in two doses) has a better side-effect profile than the Yuzpe regime and is more efficacious. However, like the Yuzpe regime it is only licensed for use within 72 hours of unprotected intercourse.

Other oral post-coital methods using the antiprogesterone mifepristone [a single dose of 600 mg (200 mg seems to be equally as effective)] or ethinylestradiol alone, also need to be administered within 72 hours of intercourse for maximum effect.

Reports have suggested that Danazol (800 mg in two doses) can be administered up to 120 hours after intercourse.

The most effective method of post-coital contraception for this woman would be to insert an intra-uterine device. I would recommend a copper one as the levonorgestrel-releasing coil (Mirena) has not been evaluated yet as a post-coital device.

Answer C2

If the missed pill had been on day 14 of the packet, I would have reassured her that she would not get pregnant provided she uses barrier methods or abstain for the next 7 days, and did not miss a further pill this cycle.

If the missed pill had been on day 20 of the packet, I would again reassure her and advise her to start the next packet immediately without the normal 7 day gap. I would also advise her to use barrier methods for the next 7 days or abstain from further acts of intercourse.

Answer C3

The Yuzpe method does not guarantee to prevent a pregnancy from occurring. Overall, it is about 98% effective if the first dose is given within 72 hours of unprotected intercourse. That means that for every 100 women that take it, two will still get pregnant. The fact that it is 80 hours after you had unprotected intercourse means that the success rate is even lower. Although I cannot quote you a figure you have a higher than 1 in 50 chance of getting pregnant even taking these tablets. Besides that, the tablets can have side effects. The commonest are nausea and vomiting, which can reduce its effectiveness even further. If you were to take the tablets and be sick you would need to come back and take two more. Breast tenderness is also a known side effect. You may also find that taking it can bring on a migraine attack, which you are already susceptible to. Your next period may be earlier or later, and you may bleed more than usual. There is also a worry that your next packet of pills may not be as effective as normal. Also, if you are worried that your husband will find out, how will you avoid intercourse for the next 7 days or explain the need for using condoms or the cap when you are already on the pill?

The coil can be inserted at any time within 5 days of unprotected intercourse. There does not appear to be any difference in its efficacy rate if it is inserted at any time during those 5 days. It is much more effective than the Yuzpe method. Many studies have shown no pregnancies when it has been used, but some have shown a pregnancy rate of about 1 in 1000 (20 times lower than if you were to take the morning after pill).

The coil does not cause you to have nausea, vomiting, breast tenderness or migraines. What your friend says is wrong. Once you have had a baby it is sometimes easier to insert a coil, and it may be less painful, but we can still fit coils in women like yourself who have never had a baby. Although we do not recommend coils as the first choice of contraception to most women who have not had a baby, there is no reason why we cannot fit one in you as a method of postcoital contraception.

The threads are very fine, like hairs, but they need to be there for us to remove the coil. We could cut the threads very short to try and stop your husband from noticing them, but I couldn't guarantee he would not find them. If you have the coil in you will not need to abstain from intercourse for 7 days or use barrier methods of contraception, so it is perhaps less likely your husband will find out.

You are correct in saying that the coil can cause heavier periods, and if we insert it today it is likely that your next period will be heavier. There is also a chance that the morning after pill could make your next period heavier. As you only need the coil in until we are sure that you are not pregnant, we could remove it without you having further heavy periods.

We know that inserting a coil carries the risk of you getting an infection in your womb. To reduce this risk I could take swabs from the neck of the womb to look for bacteria, or I could give you antibiotics. There is no evidence to suggest that coils are associated with genital warts and you need not worry about that. However, you did have unprotected intercourse with a stranger who could have warts or other sexually transmitted diseases, so you might get a further sexually transmitted disease that is nothing to do with the coil.

Answer C4

Although she could have the coil left *in situ*, the combined oral contraceptive pill still remains the best option for this woman, although the simultaneous use of condoms is highly recommended (especially with strangers) to reduce both the risks of unplanned pregnancy and sexually transmitted diseases.

Prior to fitting the coil, I would give her 500 mg of mefenamic acid orally as a premedication. When fitting a coil, I would always ask for a chaperone and ensure that there was an emergency tray containing atropine and adrenalin nearby. The first thing I would do is to ask the woman to remove her lower clothing (skirt/trousers and underwear) and lie in the dorsal position on an adjustable couch. I would cover her lower body with a sheet (or blanket) and then I would raise the couch to a comfortable height. Using sterile gloves I would perform a bimanual examination to assess the uterine size and position and exclude any uterine or adnexal tenderness.

Using a Cusco's speculum I would visualize the cervix, and carefully inspect it to ensure there was no evidence of a purulent discharge that could indicate an infection. If I was not going to 'cover' her with antibiotics, I would take high vaginal and endocervical swabs to screen for infection. I would then cleanse the cervix with a sterile cotton wool ball (held in sponge forceps and dipped in an aqueous antiseptic) to remove mucus from the external os.

As she is nulliparous I would then grasp the anterior lip of her cervix with a vulsellum, warning her that she may feel a little pinch. If she is feeling a lot of discomfort at this point I would consider injecting lignocaine for a paracervical block. I would then take a sound, dip the end into the aqueous antiseptic and gently insert it through her cervical os, in the direction of her uterus (ante or retroverted). I would warn her that she might feel some crampy abdominal pains at this time. Once I have measured the length of the uterine cavity, I would ensure that I was fitting the coil to the same length. I would load the coil into its introducer, dip it in the aqueous antiseptic and then insert it into the uterus. If necessary, I would use the smallest dilators to dilate her cervix to ensure I could fit the device. I would remove the introducer, ensuring that the coil remained *in utero* and cut the threads short with a pair of scissors. Obviously, I would stop at any point if she felt too uncomfortable. Finally, I would remove the speculum and help her to sit up. I would explain that she might get some further cramping pains (if this is the case, she should take a non-steroidal anti-inflammatory drug, e.g. mefenamic acid, ibuprofen) and some bleeding, and would provide her with a sanitary towel to wear. I would then arrange for her to have a cup of tea before sorting out a date for a follow-up visit.

I would use a copper coil, preferably a copper T (or multiload 375), depending on availability.

Answer C5

The first thing I would do is call for help. I would remove any instruments from her cervical os. I would immediately check her airway, breathing and circulation. If possible, I would tilt the couch head-down and elevate her legs. If her airway is patent, she is breathing and has a cardiac output, but remains bradycardic I would inject 0.5 mg of atropine slowly IV. If there were no evidence of a pulse, I would thump her praecordium before commencing full cardiopulmonary resuscitation.

Further reading

Cheng L, Gulmezoglu AM, Ezcurra E, Van Look PFA (2000) Interventions for emergency contraception (Cochrane Review). In: *Cochrane Library*, Issue 4. Update Software, Oxford.

Glasier A (1993) Post coital contraception. *Curr. Obstet. Gynaecol.* **3**: 91–96.

Glasier A (1995) Emergency contraception and RU 486. In: *Contraception* (Update postgraduate centre series). Reed Healthcare Communications, pp. 44–45.

Guillebaud J (1993) *Contraception: your questions answered*, 2nd edn. Churchill Livingstone, Edinburgh.

Loudon N, Glasier A, Gebbie A (eds) (1995) *Handbook of Family Planning and Reproductive Health Care*. Churchill Livingstone, Edinburgh.

Slade R *et al.* (1998) Contraception and sterilisation. In: *Key Topics in Obstetrics and Gynaecology*, 2nd edn. BIOS Scientific Publishers Ltd, Oxford, pp. 22–25.

Van Look PFA, von Hertzen H (1993) Emergency contraception. In: Drife JO, Baird DT (eds), *Contraception*. Br. Med. Bull. **49**: 158–170.

CIRCUIT 1

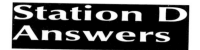

Answer D1

First, the name of the compound sounds good. It is quite authoritative, and would make you think that it would stop detrusor activity.

The language is very promotional and some of their facts sound a little unbelievable. For instance, if you quickly read the information you would think that 40% of women suffer from urge incontinence. This is a much higher incidence than has been reported elsewhere. When checking the reference, this is taken from an abstract looking at 30 pensioners, so the figure is probably unrepresentative of the population as a whole.

In the next paragraph it insinuates that Detrusorstop is the best treatment for urge incontinence and is superior to many other drugs. It refers to tests and studies and again uses strong words like 'proved', 'superior' and 'extensive'. The references that support these statements are weak; they include a case report and a pilot study. There are no references of randomized control trials to confirm it is the best, and no direct comparisons mentioned to other drugs. The references probably do not support the claim that it is the 'drug of choice'.

The graph looks impressive, but is compared to placebo and we do not know what the improvement actually means. It could be cure – no urgency or detrusor instability, or just an improvement in the length of time from desire to void to actual micturition. They also claim that this graph represents patient compliance. Again it depends on what the improvement actually means. The graph is referenced from unpublished data, using rhesus monkeys that have had Methotrexate instilled into their bladders to mimic detrusor instability. This is not the sort of data you would expect to be used to substantiate their claims, and may prove nothing.

They suggest that the drug can be commenced following an initial consultation without the need for any investigations – this should not be recommended as good practice.

Finally they say that 8 out of 10 women would prefer it, but there is no mention of sample size – they may have asked only 10 women. The word 'would' may imply that these are not women who have actually taken the drug, they just like the look of it – perhaps by being shown the graph.

Improvements would include better data (if available), numbers and details of the types of studies performed (to more accurately grade the data and evidence).

More robust data and figures should be included – for instance the incidence mentioned of 40% is too high. Some of the advice should also be clarified – for example, starting it without any investigations is not a sensible idea.

Answer D2

Evidence-based medicine is the conscientious, explicit and judicious use of current best evidence in making decisions about the care of individual patients by integrating individual clinical expertise with the best available external clinical evidence from systematic research.

It does not replace or detract from individual clinical expertise – the proficiency, judgement and surgical skill that we gain only through observation and supervised practice (Sackett *et al.*, 1996).

Answer D3

There are various levels of evidence, which differ according to its quality and applicability. The levels of evidence can be graded into five, with level I being the strongest and level V the weakest.

Level	Type of evidence
I	Strong evidence from at least one systematic review of multiple, well-designed randomized controlled trials.
II	Strong evidence from at least one properly designed randomized control trial of appropriate size.
III	Evidence from well-designed trials without randomization, single group, pre-post, cohort, time series or matched case-controlled studies.
IV	Evidence from well-designed non-experimental studies from more than one centre or research group.
V	Opinions of respected authorities, based on clinical evidence, descriptive studies or reports of expert committees.

In its guidelines, the Royal College of Obstetricians and Gynaecologists uses three levels of evidence:

Level	Type of evidence
Grade A	Randomized controlled trials (Level I & II)
Grade B	Other robust experimental or observational studies (Level III & IV)
Grade C	More limited evidence, but the advice relies on expert opinion and has the endorsement of respected authorities (Level V)

Answer D4

Randomization is the method used to divide subjects into groups; in its most simplistic form it is equivalent to the toss of a coin. In a randomized controlled trial, the participants are randomly allocated to either one intervention (e.g. experimental drug) or another (e.g. placebo). The process is designed to obtain groups that are representative of a larger population, and any differences (at inclusion) between the groups will be those due to chance alone. With regard to outcome, because the groups are identical except for the intervention, any differences should (in theory) be attributable to the intervention.

An example of a randomized controlled trial recently published is the ORACLE trial.

Randomized controlled trials are felt to be the gold standard and to provide the best evidence. They are the only way to avoid known and unknown selection biases (systematic errors) that weaken observational studies. They do not guarantee that the comparison groups are exactly matched in respect of all characteristics of prognostic importance, but do guarantee that the subjects of the comparison groups would be selected by chance rather than by any biased selection. That is why it is considered to be the methodological 'gold standard' for comparing alternative forms of care. A randomized control trial does not always guarantee the absence of selection bias unless selective recruitment into and withdrawal from the study are excluded with certainty.

Advantages are:

- Rigorous evaluation of a single variable in a precisely defined group

- Prospective design

- Seeks to falsify rather than confirm the hypothesis

- Potentially eradicates bias

- Allows for meta-analysis

Disadvantages are:

- Expensive and time consuming – often takes a long time to recruit

- Often performed on too few patients

- Failure to randomize all eligible patients

Answer D5

Bias can occur at various stages throughout a research study. Selection bias can be theoretically eliminated by randomization.

'Masking' or 'blinding' can minimize the bias that results when those receiving, providing or evaluating care know which of the alternative forms of care has been received. It is particularly useful when one or more of the forms of care is likely to have psychologically mediated (placebo) effects on the outcome of interest. It also minimizes the ability of the care-giver to adjust the remainder of their care in the light of their knowledge of the initial part of the study.

Bias may arise from the assessor's knowledge of which form of care has been received. This may be eliminated by having the outcomes assessed by independent observers, who are not aware of the forms of care allocation.

Answer D6

Random errors (the play of chance) may give misleading results despite avoiding selection biases. Random errors are reduced by increasing the sample size. Tests of significance are used to assess the likelihood of the observed differences between the alternative forms of care being a reflection of random errors.

Answer D7

True positive (TP): the test result is positive in the presence of the clinical abnormality.

True negative (TN): the test result is negative in the absence of the clinical abnormality.

False positive (FP): the test result is positive in the absence of the clinical abnormality.

False negative (FN): the test result is negative in the presence of the clinical abnormality.

Sensitivity: the proportion of all cases of the clinical abnormality that have an abnormal test result

$$TP/TP + FN$$

Specificity: the proportion of cases with no clinical abnormality that have a normal test result

$$TN/TN + FP$$

Positive predictive value: the proportion of cases with an abnormal test result that have the clinical abnormality

$$TP/TP + FP$$

Negative predictive value: the proportion of cases with a normal test result that do not have the clinical abnormality

$$TN/TN + FN$$

Relative risk: a relative risk of 1 means that the observation does not indicate a distinguished risk that is any different from the population as a whole. Above 1 the observation indicates an increased risk, below 1 a reduced risk.

$$\text{Relative risk} = \frac{TP/TP + FP}{FN/FN + TN}$$

Likelihood ratio (odds ratio): the concept is similar to that of relative risk, but combines the results of a series of tests:

$$\text{Likelihood ratio} = \frac{TP / TP + FN}{FP / FP + TN} \quad or \quad \frac{\text{Sensitivity}}{1\text{-Specificity}}$$

Receiver operating characteristics (ROC) curve: is a graph of sensitivity versus the false-positive rate.

Bayes' theorem: is a way to calculate the predictive value of test results by comparing the probability of a given abnormality *before* a test is done (the 'prior probability') with the probability of the abnormality *after* the test has been done (the 'posterior probability').

Answer D8

When evaluating a test you need to check the following.

Primary guides:

● Presence of an independent 'blind' comparison with a reference standard.

● The patient sample is representative of an appropriate spectrum of patients to whom the test would be applied in clinical practice.

Secondary guides:

● Whether the results of the test being evaluated influenced the decision to perform the reference standard.

● Whether the methods to perform the test were described in sufficient detail to permit replication.

To assess the validity of a review article, check the following:

● Did the review address a focused clinical question?

● Were appropriate inclusion criteria used to select articles?

● Were important relevant articles missed?

● Was the validity of the included studies appraised?

- Were the results of different studies similar?

- Were the assessments of the studies reproducible?

- What are the overall results of the review?

- How precise are the results?

- Were all clinically relevant outcomes considered?

- Are the results applicable to your patients?

- Do the likely treatment benefits outweigh the potential harm and costs?

Further reading

Chard T, Lilford RJ (1991) How useful is a test? In: Studd J (ed.) *Progress in Obstetrics and Gynaecology,* Vol. 9, pp. 3–15. Churchill Livingstone, Edinburgh.

Cooke IE (1996) Finding the evidence. In: Cooke IE, Sackett DL (eds), *Baillière's Clinical Obstetrics and Gynaecology International Practice and Research*, Vol. 10, Evidence-Based Obstetrics and Gynaecology, pp. 551–567. WB Saunders, London.

Crowley P (1996) Using an overview. In: Cooke IE, Sackett DL (eds), *Baillière's Clinical Obstetrics and Gynaecology International Practice and Research,* Vol. 10, Evidence-Based Obstetrics and Gynaecology, pp. 585-597. WB Saunders, London.

Deeks JJ, Morris JM (1996) Evaluating diagnostic tests. In: Cooke IE, Sackett DL (eds), *Baillière's Clinical Obstetrics and Gynaecology International Practice and Research,* Vol. 10, Evidence-Based Obstetrics and Gynaecology, pp. 613-630. WB Saunders, London.

Grant JM (1995) Randomised trials and the British Journal of Obstetrics and Gynaecology. Minimum requirements for publication. *Br. J. Obstet. Gynaecol.* **102**: 849–850.

Greenhalgh T (1997) How to read a paper: Getting your bearings (deciding what the paper is about). *Br. Med. J.* **315**: 243–246.

Jaeschke R, Guyatt G, Sackett DL (1994) Users' guides to the medical literature. III. How to use an article about a diagnostic test. A. Are the results of the study valid? *JAMA* **271**: 389–391.

Oxman AD, Cook DJ, Guyatt GH (1994) For the Evidence-Based Medicine Working Group. Users' guides to the medical literature. VI. How to use an overview. *JAMA* **272**: 1367–1371.

Sackett DL, Rosenberg WMC, Gray JAM *et al.* (1996) Evidence-based medicine: what it is and what it isn't. *Br. Med. J.* **312**: 71–72.

CIRCUIT 1

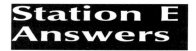

Answer E1

This does not appear to be a pregnancy-related problem. She has a negative pregnancy test, and her scan findings are consistent with ovarian inhibition secondary to the pill. Her full blood count is normal except for the mild leucocytosis. She is hyponatraemic with a raised urea and normal potassium level. Although her urea may be raised secondary to her vomiting, she would be more likely to be hypokalaemic rather than hyponatraemic. Her bilirubin and AST are markedly raised, which suggests acute hepatocellular damage. In view of these findings, the fact that she is on the pill and the history of alcohol consumption, the diagnosis is acute intermittent porphyria.

The diagnosis can be confirmed by measuring the output of urinary porphobilinogen and δ-aminolaevulinic acid, which will be increased.

Management of the acute attack would be supportive. I would refer her to the physicians. She would need careful fluid and electrolyte balance and adequate opiate analgesia. In the long term I would advise her to discontinue taking the oral contraceptive pill.

Answer E2 (i)

The likely cause is male factor, as she appears to be ovulating and has patent tubes.

I would wish to repeat his semen analysis and check his gonadotrophins.

Answer E2 (ii)

Both his semen analyses have shown azoospermia. His gonadotrophins are raised and his testosterone is low. This would suggest primary testicular failure. The commonest cause of primary testicular failure is Klinefelter's syndrome. He should be examined for gynaecomastia, a buccal smear could be taken and he should have some serum sent for chromosomal analysis.

Answer E3

The likely diagnosis is thalassaemia minor. She has a mild anaemia with a haemoglobin of 10.9 g/dl (normal = 11.5–16.5 g/dl). This is associated with low mean corpuscular volume of 62 fl (normal = 80–96 fl) and mean corpuscular haemoglobin of 22 g/dl (normal = 27–33 g/dl). A microcytic hypochromic anaemia is characteristic of either iron deficiency or thalassaemia. As her serum iron level and total iron binding capacity are within the normal range (11–30 μmol/l and 45–78 μmol/l, respectively) this would suggest thalassaemia. As her anaemia is mild, it is likely to be thalassaemia minor.

Haemoglobin electrophoresis would confirm the diagnosis, showing an increase in HbA_2.

CIRCUIT 1

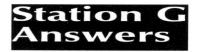

Answer G1

Her symptoms and history of gonadotrophin therapy would suggest ovarian hyper-stimulation syndrome (OHSS). The onset 4 days after embryo transfer suggests a late presentation, of mild to moderate degree.

Answer G2

GnRH analogues, gonadotrophins (FSH, human menopausal gonadotrophin, human chorionic gonadotrophin) and antiestrogens (mainly clomiphene citrate, also tamoxifen) can all cause OHSS, though the last is commonly associated only with the mild form.

There are various risk factors for the development of OHSS. Particular factors in this woman are her relatively young age, slim bodily habitus, polycystic ovaries and choice of ovulation induction agents. The combination of a GnRH analogue with hMG increases the risk. Other risk factors include previous OHSS, large numbers of follicles (and eggs recovered), and high estradiol levels on the day of hCG administration. The final risk factor is pregnancy.

Answer G3

OHSS is associated with an increase in vascular permeability, although the source of this remains unclear. This increased permeability leads to intravascular depletion as proteins leak out of the capillaries and alter the oncotic pressure. The increased vascular permeability can lead to the development of ascites, pulmonary oedema and even pericardiac oedema.

Ascites is not always diagnosed clinically, so an abdomino-pelvic ultrasound scan should be arranged. This also allows estimation of ovarian size – useful for categorizing the degree of hyperstimulation. If there was any concern about pulmonary oedema a chest X-ray should be taken.

The intravascular depletion leads to a fall in blood pressure, with consequent decreased renal perfusion and increased vascular stasis. The decreased renal perfusion results in the generation of renin from the juxta-glomerular apparatus in the kidney. This activates the angiotensin–aldosterone system to increase blood pressure (angiotensin II increases thirst and causes potent vasoconstriction; aldosterone promotes sodium resorption from the distal tubules of the nephrons). The decreased renal perfusion reduces the glomerular filtration rate (causing an increase in the serum urea and creatinine levels), decreases urinary output and stimulates the secretion of antidiuretic hormone. In turn, this will cause fluid retention leading to hyponatraemia. The reduced renal excretion will also eventually cause hyperkalaemia and the development of a metabolic acidosis.

Therefore, I would want to take blood in order to test urea and electrolyte levels and renal function. I would also want her liver function and albumin to be checked.

The intravascular stasis will promote venous (and even arterial) thrombosis; this is compounded by the haemoconcentration secondary to the intravascular depletion. Ultimately, disseminated intravascular coagulopathy may result.

Thus, I would want to carry out a full blood count (for platelets and packed cell volume) and a clotting screen.

Answer G4

Her full blood count reveals a raised packed cell volume (haematocrit). This, in combination with her hyponatraemia and elevated serum levels of urea and creatinine suggests dehydration. She is mildly hyperkalaemic. All other blood results are normal.

Her chest X-ray is unremarkable.

Her ultrasound scan confirms the presence of free fluid in her pelvis and shows that her ovaries are moderately enlarged (8–12 cm).

I would admit her to the ward. My initial management would be conservative and supportive. I would explain the diagnosis and its implications to her and her partner.

I would gain IV access and rehydrate her with normal saline (without additional potassium) at the rate of 1 l per hour.

To help with her vomiting I would prescribe an anti-emetic to be given parenterally.

If she was still suffering from pain I would prescribe simple analgesia (paracetamol, codeine). If this was insufficient I would prescribe parenteral opioids.

Thrombo-prophylaxis with TED stockings or subcutaneous heparin is important.

Her general condition needs careful monitoring. I would ask the nursing staff to take regular measurements of her abdominal girth, weight, and vital signs. I would consider catheterizing her to enable me to closely monitor her fluid balance.

I would want to repeat her blood tests later.

Answer G5

Her symptoms suggest hypovolaemic shock, ascites and possibly the development of pleural effusions.

She is now becoming severely dehydrated and haemoconcentrated; her white cell count is elevated. She is polycythaemic secondary to dehydration (high Hb) and her packed cell volume is significantly raised. Her hyponatraemia has worsened and her renal function is deteriorating with further rises in her urea and creatinine. Her potassium level also continues to climb. The increased vascular permeability has now resulted in a fall in her albumin level, which would decrease the colloid osmotic pressure still further compounding the intravascular depletion.

Her clotting screen is now prolonged and her platelets are beginning to fall suggesting the onset of disseminated intravascular coagulation.

Her liver function tests are mildly raised.

The results and her symptoms suggest a deterioration of her condition to severe OHSS. The diagnosis of severe OHSS should be based on the following criteria: hypovolaemia (tachycardia, hypotension, decreased CVP), haemoconcentration (PCV >45%, WBC >15 x 10^9/l), generalized oedema, ascites extending to the upper abdomen, hydrothorax, oliguria (with low serum sodium and high potassium concentrations, acidosis), ovarian size >12 cm.

The patient now needs transfer to a high dependency unit, with management by a multidisciplinary team as it could be life threatening. She will need a CVP line inserting and if her condition deteriorates further she is at risk of developing adult respiratory distress syndrome or suffering a cardiorespiratory arrest.

Appropriate opioid analgesia should be given.

Simultaneous intravenous albumin and crystalloid infusions should be used to treat her hypovolaemic shock, while carefully monitoring vital signs, CVP and fluid balance. Diuretics should not be used until her hypovolaemia is corrected. Dialysis should be considered if her renal function deteriorates further.

If not already commenced, prophylactic heparin should be administered together with the TED stockings.

Paracentesis and a pleural tap should be considered to alleviate her dyspnoea (bearing in mind that this removes protein-rich fluid from the body and needs replacing).

If a pregnancy was confirmed, after counselling, withdrawal of luteal support, and in critical cases, termination of pregnancy should be considered.

Surgery is only necessary if internal bleeding or ovarian torsion or rupture occurs and should only be performed by an experienced surgeon, as the ovaries are very fragile.

Answer G6

Patients at risk (PCOS, previous OHSS) should be identified prior to ovulation induction. However, it should be remembered that these factors are less sensitive in predicting the late form of OHSS. Low risk methods of the ovulation induction should be employed first:

- anti-estrogens;

- laparoscopic ovarian drilling;

- gonadotrophin without GnRH analogues;

- FSH rather than hMG.

If multiple small follicles are present early on in the cycle, this can act as a risk factor. High estradiol levels on the day of the hCG trigger (>6000) and more than 30 oocytes retrieved predict the development of OHSS. All follicles should be aspirated to try and reduce the risk.

'Step down' regimes have been developed where the initial doses of FSH are reduced as the cycle progresses. They are adjusted in accordance with estradiol levels and the number of developing follicles. This is a more physiological regime and is associated with lower risks for the development of OHSS.

If early OHSS has occurred, the embryos should be frozen and the cycle cancelled to avoid late OHSS. After embryo transfer, withdrawal of hCG support or converting to progesterone (cyclogest PR/PV) should be considered.

Patient education and proper counselling at the initial visit, about the risk and early symptoms of OHSS is important, as well as supplying them with a contact telephone number with 24 hour access.

A number of preventive methods (intravenous albumin infusion at the time of oocyte recovery, ACE inhibitors) are currently under evaluation.

Further reading

Amso NN, Shaw RW (1997) OHSS assisted reproduction treatment. In: Shaw RW, Soutter WP, Stanton SL (eds), *Gynaecology,* pp. 281–302. Churchill Livingstone, Edinburgh.

Balen AH, Jacobs HS (1997) *Infertility in Practice,* pp. 309–329. Churchill Livingstone, Edinburgh.

Jenkins J, Mathur R (1998) Ovarian hyper-stimulation syndrome. PACE Review No 98/06.

Mathur RS, Joels LA, Akande AV, Jenkins JM (1996) The prevention of ovarian hyperstimulation syndrome. *Br. J. Obstet. Gynaecol.* **103**: 740–746.

Royal College of Obstetricians and Gynaecologists (1995) Management and prevention of ovarian hyperstimulation syndrome (OHSS). RCOG Guideline No. 5. Royal College of Obstetricians and Gynaecologists, London.

CIRCUIT 1

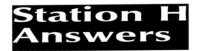

Answer H1

I would introduce myself, take a history and examine her abdomen. I would explain initially what is meant by the term 'breech', the fact that it occurs in 3–4% of pregnancies at term, and the implications if it is confirmed. Although many breeches can be detected clinically, I would want to arrange to scan her to confirm the presentation. I would also like the scan to be able to define the type of breech (extended, flexed or footling), the attitude of the fetal head, estimate the fetal weight and to rule out any fetal or pelvic abnormalities.

Answer H2

Initially, I would discuss the scan findings with her – in this case, an appropriately grown baby with its legs extended so that its feet are pointing towards its face. I would tell her that the placenta is on the back wall of the womb and that there are no obvious reasons for this baby to be breech.

I would try to reassure her that the baby might turn by itself and would then discuss vaginal delivery. I would begin by explaining the results of the randomized trial for the delivery of term breeches. This was the largest study of its kind to ever have taken place, and was designed to answer the question of which method of delivery (vaginal or caesarean section) is the safest way to deliver breech babies like hers. The study included 121 centres around the world, and involved in excess of 2000 women. It concluded that there is good scientific evidence to confirm that average-sized term babies delivered via caesarean section have a better short-term outcome than those delivered vaginally. The study showed that there were more problems and deaths in those babies born vaginally when compared to those born by caesarean section (3.3% vs. 1.3%), and there was no significant difference to the mother whichever way she was delivered. I would stress that there is still debate about the long-term outcome of breech babies when compared with those delivered head first, and that studies are ongoing. I would mention the worrying results of one study that showed that almost 1 in 5 breech babies will suffer a handicap or other health problems, regardless of the mode of delivery.

Following the results of the term breech trial I would recommend an operative rather than vaginal delivery if the baby remained as breech, but I would agree that ultimately the decision was hers.

If she insisted on a trial of vaginal delivery, I would go on to discuss the importance of the appropriate selection of cases for vaginal delivery, bearing in mind the type of breech (flexed or extended), fetal attitude (no hyperextension of the fetal head), signs of potential feto-pelvic disproportion (estimated fetal weight >4 kg), pelvic or fetal abnormalities, etc. These factors become largely irrelevant for caesarean section.

Caesarean section is indicated when the risks of feto-pelvic disproportion, cord prolapse or fetal distress in labour are high. There is no evidence to suggest that pelvimetry is of any benefit in assessing adequate pelvic size clinical judgement is satisfactory.

I would explain that vaginal delivery can be safe, was previously thought to be associated with lower maternal risks and a shorter hospital stay. The risk of fetal trauma (occipital diasthesis, intra-/peri-ventricular haemorrhage, generalized bruising), however, is higher. Therefore, I would explain the need for continuous monitoring in labour with a CTG, the possibility of performing an FBS (via the buttocks) if monitoring suggested compromise. I would discuss regional analgesia and the actual delivery – the need for an IVI, an episiotomy, and delivery (in the lithotomy position) to be conducted or supervised by a senior and experienced doctor. I would inform her of my wish to have a paediatrician present at the delivery. I would also explain that the need for a caesarean section could not be ruled out even if she insisted on a trial of labour.

I would inform her also of the complications that can be associated with a vaginal breech delivery – higher rates of cord prolapse, head entrapment from an undilated cervix, and difficult delivery of the head.

I would also convey to her the fact that there is little information available to confirm or deny the safety of augmenting labour with syntocinon, or inducing labour if necessary.

Finally, I would agree that the decision to have a vaginal delivery is hers, providing the situation does not alter significantly between now and the onset of labour.

Answer H3

The chances of the baby turning to a head presentation at this stage would be small. There are some people who advocate adopting the knee–chest position for 15 minutes every 2 hours throughout the day (Elkin's manoeuvre), although some small randomized trials have not confirmed that this works. Success rates of spontaneous version of up to 90% have been reported.

The only thing that I could do to help would be to attempt an ECV. ECV at term reduces the incidence of caesarean section by 50%. As she is Nigerian she should have a higher chance of success with this process (93% for black African women compared to 48% for the UK population). I would outline the risks and the procedure, and advise her that the careful selection of cases is necessary to try to ensure success. The procedure may be technically more difficult in primigravidae, when the fetal back is posterior, the fetal legs are extended and the presenting part is engaged. Other factors associated with failure are abnormal liquor volume, an anterior placenta and significant maternal obesity. There is an association between the success rate and the obstetrician's skills. If the version was unsuccessful it could be repeated and would not stop a trial of vaginal delivery. On the other hand, successful version does not guarantee avoidance of a section.

Answer H4

I would perform the ECV with the woman awake, with facilities for emergency delivery nearby. Fetal wellbeing should be assessed with a CTG for 20 minutes before (and after) the procedure. I would personally scan her (or arrange a scan) before the ECV to check the position, confirm adequate liquor volume and possibly exclude a cord around the baby.

Following the CTG and scan, I would ask her to empty her bladder and then lie on a bed, with a mild degree of head-down tilt. Aorto-caval compression should be avoided by lateral tilt. I would commence an intravenous infusion of a tocolytic (e.g. ritodrine 50 μg/min in 5% dextrose), which has been proved to be effective in increasing success.

Standing on the right-hand side of the woman, I would disengage the breech from the pelvis with my right hand. I would place my left hand over the head and then begin to rotate the baby by applying inequal pressure simultaneously with both hands, but in opposite directions. The left hand should really only steady the head, with most force applied to the breech. This will reduce the potential risk of neck injuries. The direction of rotation depends on the position of the fetal back – the direction being that which promotes flexion of the head. The process should occur with continuous and constant force, and although it may feel uncomfortable, it should not cause pain. Severe pain or vaginal bleeding would be an indication to stop, as would not achieving version after 5 minutes. Following the attempt I would perform a scan to confirm version, discontinue the tocolytic and repeat the CTG. I would keep the woman in for at least half an hour, and then arrange to see her 1 week later.

All Rhesus-negative women should have Anti-D 500 IU given and a Kleihauer test performed.

Further reading
Enkin M, Keirse MJNC, Renfrew M, Neilson J (1996) *A Guide To Effective Care In Pregnancy and Childbirth,* 2nd edn. Oxford University Press, Oxford.

Hannah ME, Hannah WJ, Hewson SA *et al.* (2000) Planned caesarean section versus planned vaginal birth for breech presentation at term: a randomised multicentre trial. *Lancet* **356**: 1375–1383.

Lindquist A, Norden-Lindeberg S, Hanson U (1997) Perinatal mortality and route of delivery in term breech presentations. *Br. J. Obstet. Gynaecol.* **104**: 1288–1291.

Myerscough P (1998) The practice of external cephalic version. *Br. J. Obstet. Gynaecol.* **105**: 1043–1045.

Royal College of Obstetrics and Gynaecology (1999) The management of breech presentation. RCOG Guideline No. 20.

Slade R, *et al.* (1998) Key Topics in Obstetrics and Gynaecolgy, 2nd edn, pp. 175–178.

CIRCUIT 1

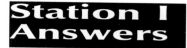

Answer I1

I would explain to her that she has a 'prolapse' of the uterus and the bladder. This means that her uterus is coming down into her vagina, and her bladder is bulging through the front wall of the vagina. The stress incontinence she complains of may be caused by descent of the bladder neck (which controls continence) due to weakness of its supports. The usual causes of weakness of the supports of the uterus and bladder are congenital or developmental, trauma and denervation during childbirth, and laxity of vaginal fascia after the menopause due to loss of the perivaginal venous plexus as a consequence of estrogen deficiency. Chronic cough, constipation, obesity and heavy weight lifting exacerbate the problem by increasing intra-abdominal pressure. It is important to solve these problems, if they are present, before embarking on any treatment.

The treatment options would depend on how debilitating she considers the symptoms to be, and whether she wishes conservative or surgical treatment. I would explain that there are no medical treatments for this condition and its natural history is to worsen if untreated. I would discuss referral to a physiotherapist for pelvic floor exercises, inserting a ring pessary or performing a vaginal hysterectomy with repair of the bladder support (anterior colporrhaphy).

A pessary could be inserted to rectify the prolapse. This is a large ring that sits at the back of the vagina to keep the uterus pushed up, but it is a temporary measure and the pessary needs to be reinserted at regular intervals of 4–6 months, depending on the type of the pessary (shelf or ring pessary). The side effects are excessive vaginal discharge, vaginal infection and ulcer.

Physiotherapy is not usually effective in postmenopausal prolapse, but it could be used as an adjunctive with other treatments.

Vaginal hysterectomy with anterior colporrhaphy is a curative treatment for the prolapse, though there is a chance of vaginal vault prolapse occurring at a later date in 2% of cases. Repair of the bladder support could make the incontinence worse as it corrects the kink at the bladder neck. To reduce the chance of this problem, a suture is placed around the bladder neck to improve its support (suburethral buttressing). The stitches under the bladder will cure stress incontinence in about 50% of women; the others may need further surgery. It is a major operation and can be associated with complications such as excessive bleeding; injury to the bladder, ureter and bowel; urinary tract, wound and chest infections; and clots in the leg veins and lungs. The postoperative hospital stay is usually 3–4 days and the recovery period is about 3–4 weeks. Topical estrogen cream may be used for 2 weeks before the operation to improve vaginal atrophy if it is present.

Answer 12

I would check her full blood count and urea and electrolytes (on frusemide). I would arrange for a chest X-ray and ECG (hypertensive) to be performed. I would also arrange for an X-ray of her cervical spine (rheumatoid arthritis). I would arrange for a check up in the preoperative clinic and by the anaesthetist. I would also check that she has a recent negative cervical smear.

(Many would argue that urodynamics should be undertaken before surgery is contemplated.)

Answer 13

I would discuss this with the woman and take her wishes into consideration. If she had no strong feelings about removal I would check them during the operation, and if they looked normal I would leave them. Although it is possible to remove ovaries during vaginal hysterectomy in 95–99% cases, their removal increases the operative time and the chance of bleeding, while the chance of ovarian cancer developing would be minimal.

If she wished that they were removed, I would aim to do this vaginally after removal of her uterus, providing they were mobile. Having clamped the infundibulopelvic and round ligaments together, I would tie the round ligaments separately. Using a curved clamp (Babcock or ovum forceps are alternatives), I would grasp the fallopian tube and pull this down until I could reach the ovary. I would then safely place a clamp behind the ovary before dividing the vessels.

If the ovaries were immobile, or as an alternative approach, they could be removed laparoscopically either initially or once the vaginal vault was closed.

Answer 14

The options for vault prolapse would be operative correction or insertion of a pessary. The former is the better option.

There are several surgical techniques to correct vault prolapse, such as colporrhaphy; transvaginal sacrospinous colpopexy, abdominal sacro-colpopexy, abdominoperineal technique and colpocleisis, vaginectomy and colpotomy. The last operations are appropriate in sexually inactive women in whom other procedures are considered inappropriate or have failed.

Colporrhaphy in the form of an anterior and posterior vaginal repair with a McCall-type posterior culdoplasty has been the usual operation for vault prolapse. This procedure often results in a short, narrow vagina. This is also less effective as the uterosacral ligaments are likely to be attenuated and difficult to identify in women with vault prolapse, thus unlikely to provide adequate and sustained support to the vaginal vault.

Abdominal sacro-colpopexy, by open procedure or by laparoscopy, is effective in more than 90% of cases. The procedure involves suspending the vaginal vault from the sacral promontory or hollow of the sacrum with rectus sheath or synthetic (prolene) mesh strips. The posterior pelvic peritoneum is closed over the strips, thus obliterating the pouch of Douglas. The major drawback is the use of the abdominal approach. The presence of a cystocele or rectocele requires an additional vaginal procedure. Intraoperative haemorrhage due to trauma to the venous plexus on the anterior aspect of the sacrum, and infection of the synthetic mesh resulting in its removal are the major complications. Elderly and obese women are not well suited to the abdominal approach.

Transvaginal sacrospinous colpopexy is the most popular method at present. The success rate is more than 95%. The vaginal vault is fixed to one of the sacrospinous ligaments with two prolene sutures. Excessive haemorrhage or nerve or rectal damage are rarely reported. This procedure is well suited to elderly and obese women. It avoids major abdominal surgery and a coexisting cystocele or rectocele can be corrected during the procedure.

Answer I5

At vaginal hysterectomy, shortening the uterosacral and cardinal ligaments, attaching them to the vaginal vault and obliteration of any enterocele sac may improve the support. In some women, sacrospinous colpopexy may be performed in addition. At abdominal hysterectomy, intrafascial hysterectomy would minimize damage to the paracolpium fibres and Moscowitz or Halban procedures may be performed to obliterate the pouch of Douglas (especially with colposuspension).

Further reading

Cardozo L (1995) Prolapse. In: Whitfield CR (ed.), *Dewhurst's Textbook of Obstetrics and Gynaecology for Postgraduates*, 5th edn, pp. 642–652. Blackwell Scientific Publications Ltd, Oxford.

Carry MP, Slack MC (1994) Vaginal vault prolapse. *Br. J. Hosp. Med.* **51**: 417–420.

Shrotri MS, Hershman MJ, Farquharson RG (1997) How to do it in surgery: laparoscopic sacral colpopexy. *Br. J. Hosp. Med.* **57**: 514–516.

Slade R. *et al.* (1998) Genital prolapse. *Key Topics in Obstetrics and Gynaecology*, 2nd edn, pp. 41–43.

CIRCUIT 1

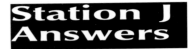

Station J
Answers

Answer J1

In view of her history of irregular vaginal bleeding and abdominal pain I would be concerned that she might have an ectopic pregnancy. The presence of the copper IUCD is a risk factor for an ectopic pregnancy. Although you could advise her to wait until the morning for a scan, or come in immediately if the pain or bleeding got worse, I would be concerned for her because she lives alone with her daughter.

Despite the fact that there are no beds in the hospital, I would ask the GP to send her to casualty from where I would arrange to scan her. My future management would then depend on the results of the scan.

Answer J2

An early intrauterine pregnancy is classically characterized by the double ring sign (formed by the true gestation sac surrounded by decidua vera and the adjacent decidua capsularis), or the eccentric location of the true sac and presence of a yolk sac. A tubal pregnancy is characterized by a well-differentiated tubal ring (doughnut or bagel sign) or a poorly differentiated tubal ring with free fluid in pouch of Douglas.

In counselling the woman I would begin by informing her that the scan confirms that she is pregnant because a very small amount of fluid (probably a pregnancy sac) has been seen in her uterus (equivalent to a pregnancy of under 5 weeks). Despite this, the exact location and viability of the pregnancy is still not clear, the reason being that the detection of a fetal pole, and preferably a fetal heart beat, is necessary to make an accurate diagnosis of a viable intrauterine pregnancy and it is too early to detect these at present. Although the scan suggests fluid within her uterus, this does not always indicate that the fetus is growing inside the uterus. Sometimes you can get these changes when there is a pregnancy outside the uterus (an ectopic pregnancy), and she will need careful monitoring over the next few weeks to distinguish what is happening in her particular case.

I would also explain to her that if the pregnancy is in her uterus and is viable, then I would recommend removing her coil. Although coil removal is associated with a risk of miscarriage, the risk is higher if the coil is left in. I would advise her that if the pregnancy appeared to be outside the uterus, it may not be safe to leave it there and she has a high chance of needing surgery.

My management would then be expectant, by monitoring her quantitative serum beta hCG levels and repeating her scan. I would take a sample of blood at that time and arrange a further sample 48 hours later. I would then observe the rate of its change (in a normal pregnancy the level should rise by more than 66%). I would also arrange a repeat high resolution transvaginal ultrasound scan a week later. If the pregnancy was viable and intrauterine I would then expect to see a fetal pole and the fetal heart beat.

Although initial monitoring with the quantitative beta hCG is safer to perform on an in-patient basis (with discharge from the hospital only after an adequte rise of the beta hCG has been demonstrated and the woman has been shown to be asymptomatic), I would consider allowing her to be treated as an outpatient. I would only consider this if she agreed to return immediately if the pain or bleeding got worse, if she developed any shoulder or neck pain, or was worried in any way.

Answer J3

The disadvantages of a laparoscopy at this point are two-fold.

With regard to specific disadvantages, at this time in the pregnancy there is a risk of missing a very early ectopic pregnancy due to its small size and disturbing an early intrauterine pregnancy if the intrauterine manipulation becomes necessary to achieve good visualization of the fallopian tubes. There is also the theoretical risk of harm to the fetus from the drugs used peri- and postoperatively.

Any laparoscopy involves risks. These may be due to the general anaesthetic or secondary to the surgery – either directly or indirectly. The introduction of the pneumoperitoneum and subsequent insertion of the trochar are associated with visceral (bladder, small and large bowel etc.), and vascular (aorta, iliac vessels etc.) damage. There is also a small risk of carbon dioxide embolism. Any of these complications may result in a laparotomy with significant morbidity and occasional mortality. Other risks include infection, thromboembolism and incisional hernias.

Answer J4

Both medical and surgical options should be considered.

Medical options include the systemic administration (intramuscularly, intra-venously or orally) of methotrexate (50 mg/m^2 of the body surface area) or its local injection directly into the gestational sac under ultrasound or laparoscopic guidance. Other substances used for the direct injection into the gestation sac include potassium chloride, hyperosmolar glucose solution and prostaglandin F$_2\alpha$. Most work has been done with methotrexate. The subsequent monitoring of the serum beta hCG level is essential to ensure adequate treatment with declining serum levels. Methotrexate might be an option here as the ectopic is unruptured, no fetal heart activity has been demonstrated, there is a small amount of fluid in the pouch of Douglas, and the serum beta hCG level is well below 10 000 IU.

Surgical management options include salpingotomy or partial/total salpingect-omy. This should be performed laparoscopically (provided adequate equipment and training). In view of the fact that her other tube is normal, I would perform a left salpingectomy rather than salpingotomy. The reason for this is that the success rates (of intrauterine pregnancies) are similar with both techniques, but persistent trophoblastic activity and future ectopic rates are lower if a salpingectomy has been performed.

Answer J5

The woman should be told that this ectopic pregnancy will have little influence on her future fecundity, but the chance of an ectopic pregnancy recurring in the future is about 10%. Therefore, I would advise that when a future pregnancy is suspected, this should be confirmed by an early pregnancy test and, if positive, an early pelvic ultrasound scan should be arranged to detect its location.

Both copper IUCDs and progesterone only contraception are best avoided as they may further increase the risk of an ectopic pregnancy. However, results seem favourable with the progestogen releasing (Mirena) coil. The combined contraceptive pill is not advisable either in view of her smoking and the side effects she has experienced previously. In view of her age and lack of partner I would also disuade her from a sterilization. Thus, barrier methods of contraception or a Mirena coil can be recommended. These methods may also confer some protection against pelvic inflammatory disease – a worry as she only has one tube remaining.

Further reading
(1999) Management of ectopic pregnancy. *Drugs Ther. Bull.* **37**: 44–46.
Mascarenhas L (1997) Ectopic pregnancy. RCOG PACE Review No. 97/07.
Mascarenhas L, Williamson J, Smith S (1997) The changing face of ectopic pregnancy. *Br. Med. J.* **315**: 141.
Royal College of Obstetricians and Gynaecologists (1999) The Management of Tubal Pregnancies. RCOG Guideline No. 21.
Slade R. *et al.* (1998) Ectopic pregnancy. In: *Key Topics in Obstetrics and Gynaecology*, 2nd edn. BIOS Scientific Publishers Ltd, Oxford.
Yao M, Tulandi T (1997) Current status of surgical and nonsurgical management of ectopic pregnancy. *Fertil. Steril.* **67**: 421–433

CIRCUIT 2

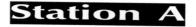

Question A1

A 53-year-old shop assistant has been referred by her GP to the gynaecological outpatients clinic. She presented to her 3 months ago complaining of hot flushes, night sweats and mood swings. She feels that these symptoms have left her unable to sleep; consequently she is feeling constantly tired. She has also noticed that her weight is increasing and she is feeling weepy and depressed. She has lost all interest in sexual intercourse. Her last menstrual period was 7 months ago, and prior to that her periods were heavy and irregular. She had two normal deliveries in the past and no previous gynaecological problems. Her contraceptive needs were met until recently by the progesterone only pill, which she has now discontinued. Her cervical smears have always been normal, as was a recent mammogram. Currently she is taking anti-hypertensive medication (her blood pressure is well controlled) and she is otherwise well. She does not smoke or drink alcohol and is not overweight. Examination is unremarkable.

Her GP has performed some blood tests and you have to ring for the results. These are:

FSH	34 IU/l
LH	18 IU/l
Estradiol	100 pmol/l
TSH	27 mU/l
T4	50 nmol/l

She wishes help for her symptoms, but following a recent television programme is worried about the risks of venous thrombosis associated with hormone replacement therapy.

What would be your initial management?

Your answer here ....

Your answer here (cont.) ....

Question A2

She returns for review in 3 months' time. She has seen Dr Hormoans, the endocrinologist, who agreed with your diagnosis of hypothyroidism. She is now taking thyroxine 100 µg per day. Although her weight has slightly reduced, her other symptoms have persisted, especially the loss of libido and hot flushes, that are 'most troublesome'. She has not had any further bleeding and is using condoms for contraception.

You feel she would benefit from a trial of HRT. Which HRT would you suggest to this woman and why?

Your answer here ....

Question A3

After appropriate counselling about the risks and benefits of HRT, the woman was commenced on an oral cyclical preparation containing 1 mg estradiol valerate and 1 mg of norethisterone (days 16–28), causing monthly withdrawal bleeds. She was discharged back to her GP who arranged a subsequent review. She attended the surgery 4 months later feeling much better. Her hot flushes had improved, as had her interest in intercourse. Her only concern was of irregular vaginal bleeding with only a small amount of loss.

How common is this problem? What are the causes of irregular bleeding and which investigations would you arrange?

Your answer here ....

Question A4

You arrange to see this woman again and perform an ultrasound and a pipelle biopsy. The woman has an ultrasound scan, which reveals her endometrium is 5 mm thick, the ovaries are atrophic and there is a small 3 cm fibroid anteriorly. The pipelle biopsy shows hyperplastic endometrium without atypia and no secretory changes. She returns to see you for the results, and during the consultation she remarks that the hot flushes, night sweats and mood swings have recurred and she is getting headaches, bloating, acne and breast tenderness when she was taking the dark (progestogen-containing) tablets. The headaches were so bad that she wished to stop taking the HRT.

What would you say with regard to her histology and which therapeutical options of management should be considered for this woman?

Your answer here ....

Question A5

The woman preferred to avoid an operation, if at all possible, and was not keen on taking extra pills or having a coil fitted. Therefore, she was started on Tibolone. Four months later she returns to the clinic with recurrent vaginal bleeding.

What would your advice be now?

Your answer here ....

Question A6

Yesterday the woman underwent a vaginal hysterectomy with bilateral salpingo-oophorectomy and she is due to commence an oestrogen-only HRT. She is interested to know when she should start the HRT, which preparation are you going to try, how long she should stay on it for and what are the potential risks for her?

Your answer here ....

Question B1

You are second on-call (specialist registrar) covering the labour ward over a weekend. You are the most senior obstetrician in the hospital. Your consultant has done his rounds and as labour ward had no problems, has gone to play golf. You are eating your lunch in the canteen when a midwife calls you to see a woman who had a normal vaginal delivery about 5 minutes ago and is now bleeding heavily.

Describe how you would manage the situation, both immediately overall and for each specific cause of a post partum haemorrhage.

Your answer here ....

Question B2

Despite your prompt arrival on labour ward and initial resuscitation, the woman's condition is deteriorating. Over the last hour and a half, since delivery she has lost at least 1000 ml of blood and her blood pressure is falling. The senior midwife has checked the placenta to ensure it was complete, you have examined her and found no lower genital tract trauma except for a small graze on her labia which is not bleeding. Her uterus remains atonic despite Syntometrine, an oxytocin infusion and bimanual compression. You have given her a total of 1 mg of prostaglandin F_2 (Hemabate) with little effect. Despite several attempts you have been unable to contact your consultant by telephone. The laboratory has been on the telephone to say that her blood group is AB negative and she has anti-Kell antibodies. They are reluctant to cross-match unless she really needs the blood. You note that her blood is now very watery.

Her blood results immediately post delivery were:

Hb	11.2 g/dl
WCC	15.2 × 10⁹/l
Plts	158 × 10⁹/l
PT	12 seconds
APTT	42 seconds
Na	134 mmol/l
K	3.2 mmol/1
U	4.7 mmol/l

What would you do next? Is there anything before a laparotomy?

Your answer here ....

Question B3

The consultant anaesthetist arrives in theatre with the news that they have contacted one of the consultant obstetricians who is not on call and is operating privately 5 miles away. Her instructions over the phone are to do what is necessary, and as soon as she has finished her hysterectomy she will come across.

You have tried to stop the bleeding by inserting a Foley catheter into the uterus but this has failed.

The estimated blood loss is now 2500 ml and replacement has started with un-crossmatched blood – she has had three units so far.

Her repeat blood results are:

Hb	5.2 g/dl
WCC	$18.6 \times 10^9/l$
Plts	$38 \times 10^9/l$
PT	24 seconds
APTT	48 seconds
Na	130 mmol/l
K	3.0 mmol/l
U	9.7 mmol/l

The consultant anaesthetist suggests you proceed before the woman exsanguinates. What would you do now?

Your answer here ....

Question B4

After the event what would you do?

Your answer here ....

Question B5

Suppose you encounter severe bleeding during a caesarean section. Is there any other method to control the bleeding besides those you have mentioned, and can you describe it?

Your answer here .. ..

CIRCUIT 2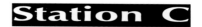

Before completing the following station, imagine this as a rest station. You have been asked to design a consent form as part of an integrated care pathway (ICP) being designed for routine sterilization operations in your hospital – The Last Chance NHS Trust. The idea of this ICP is to streamline the paperwork and reduce medical litigation. Bring your consent form with you to the next station.

Take 15 minutes to design this then proceed.

Question C1

What do you understand by the term consent? Who can give it and take it?

Your answer here ....

Question C2

What type of consents do you understand, and is written consent essential?

Your answer here ....

Question C3

When can you treat a patient without informed consent?

Your answer here ....

Question C4

What factors would you consider to decide on the options as being in the best interests of a patient who lacks the capacity to decide?

Your answer here ....

Question C5

You have come to the gynaecological ward to see a patient the day before her major operation. She was consented 2 months before in the clinic. What would you do?

Your answer here ....

CIRCUIT 2

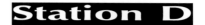

Question D1

A community midwife telephones you in the antenatal clinic from the home of Mrs Park, a young woman whom she is visiting. The woman is currently 12 weeks pregnant in her second pregnancy, and she is booking her for shared antenatal care. Mrs Park is extremely anxious. She told the community midwife that 3 days ago she spent the morning visiting a friend, whose little boy had played with her 2-year-old daughter. Later that same day, the friend's 3-year-old son developed a rash and has just been diagnosed as having chickenpox. Mrs Park cannot recall having ever had chickenpox herself, and was certainly never immunised against it. Apart from a headache, she is otherwise well, but is concerned that this might be the start of the infection and is extremely worried both for herself and for her unborn baby.

The midwife asks for your opinion as to the risk of her patient contracting chickenpox, and what should she do next.

Your answer here ....

Question D2

The midwife takes her booking bloods and asks for the Varicella zoster levels to be checked. One week later the results arrive in the antenatal clinic, where you have arranged to see Mrs Park following a dating scan. Her booking scan confirms a single viable intrauterine pregnancy consistent with her dates. She remains extremely anxious about the risks to herself and her baby of developing chickenpox.

These are the results of her viral screen. Explain the results to Mrs Park. Can you relieve her anxiety? Discuss the potential maternal and fetal risks involved and what should be done next.

NB. Assume that the diagnosis of chickenpox has been confirmed in the friend's son.

Your answer here ....

Question D3

You advise Mrs Park to have zoster immune globulin (ZiG). She wishes to know how effective it is and whether or not there are any risks associated with it.

Your answer here ....

Question D4

Mrs Park has her ZIG and you arrange to re-check her bloods for Varicella zoster antibodies. These results come back:

CENTRAL VIROLOGY LABORATORY

Mrs A. Park
Unit Number: 192076   D.O.B: 11 / 2 / 1973

Details: 12 weeks pregnant. VZ exposure.

Hepatitis B antibodies – not detected
HIV antibody   – not detected
Rubella antibody   – not detected

Varicella zoster IgG   – not detected
Varicella zoster IgM   – not detected

What does this imply?

Your answer here ....

Question D5

What would you have advised if these results had come back?

CENTRAL VIROLOGY LABORATORY
Mrs A. Park Unit Number: 192076   D.O.B: 11 / 2 / 1973
Details: 13.5 weeks pregnant. VZ exposure. **Varicella zoster IgG** – **positive** **Varicella zoster IgM** – **not detected**

Your answer here ....

Question D6

Like rubella, should we routinely screen for Varicella zoster?

Your answer here ....

Mrs Thompson, a 40-year-old woman, has come to Dr Smith's gynaecology clinic requesting a hysterectomy for heavy periods. She has been suffering from regular heavy periods for the last 2 years, since she was sterilized. A pelvic ultrasound scan done 1 month ago by her GP did not reveal any pelvic pathology. She has had medical treatment in the form of mefenamic acid, tranexamic acid and progestogens without much benefit. Her GP is now following the locally agreed guidelines and has referred her for consideration for surgery. She is fed up and wants to have a hysterectomy to get rid of the problem permanently. She has three living children, all of whom were delivered normally. She has never had an abnormal smear, smokes 20 cigarettes per day and is otherwise well. Counsel her as Dr Pepper her specialist registrar.

[This is a role-playing station, set as a simulated sequence of questions and answers in the gynaecology clinic. Try and answer fully all Mrs Thompson's questions and concerns. Begin as if you were meeting Mrs Thompson for the first time. Her responses are in bold. Ask a friend to role play this Station by reading out the bold type.]

Hello, Mrs Thompson I am Dr Pepper, I work with Dr Smith and I am her registrar. Can I check your name and date of birth please?

Hello, I am Mrs Pamela Thompson. My date of birth is 18th September 1961.

The letter from your doctor says that you would like a hysterectomy.

Yes. I want a permanent cure for these wretched periods. I have tried everything, but nothing seems to be working, and they are ruining my life. Each month when I am on, I can't leave the house for 2 days. Last month the clots were so bad that I had to sleep on a plastic sheet. Our family is complete and I have been sterilized. I have discussed it with my husband and my doctor, and it seems that hysterectomy is the only solution.

You are correct, but hysterectomy is not the only cure. There are alternative forms of surgery and some medical treatments that you may not have tried. You are suffering from a very common condition and it isn't life threatening, so there are alternatives to hysterectomy. I know your doctor has tried you on most, but not all tablets. The oral contraceptive pill often works well to control bleeding by giving you a controlled cycle, but you would be better to stop smoking if we tried this. Another alternative would be to give you an injection to switch off your pituitary gland (GnRHa). The pituitary gland sends signals to stimulate the ovaries, and the injection makes you menopausal, so we could give you HRT at the same time. This might make you bleed irregularly and is a long-term therapy. Alternatively, has your doctor talked to you about the Mirena coil?

No.
There is a new type of coil called the Mirena, which is very effective in reducing the blood loss in women with heavy periods. It releases one type of the hormone progesterone constantly for 5 years. When your body is exposed to a progestogen continuously it makes the womb 'think' that you are pregnant. This makes the lining of the womb thin and dramatically reduces the amount of blood lost. It does not stop you from ovulating, but does prevent menstruation. Within 3 months of having this inserted it will reduce the blood loss by 85% and this decreases by 97% after 1 year of use. We actually find that after 1 year of use over a third of women will not have any further bleeding at all.

No treatment is without side effects, so what are the unwanted effects of Mirena?

The biggest problem is that they cause irregular bleeding. This tends to be spotting and settles down with time, but you may have to persevere for the first few months. Other effects are normally minimal and are hormonal, such as mood changes, headache, breast tenderness, nausea, acne and hair growth. Although it doesn't normally interfere with ovulation there is a risk of (functional) ovarian cysts developing. These can be unnoticed or may cause pain. The coil can be expelled and there are risks of introducing infection and perforating your uterus during fitting but these are very uncommon.

You mentioned that there are other surgical treatments – are those the laser ones I've read about in women's magazines?

Yes, there is also an operation called an endometrial resection or ablation, where we destroy the lining of the uterus. Resection means cutting away the lining of the womb, ablation means destroying it. Overall, it is effective in 80% of cases over a period of 3 years. In about one third of women, it stops their periods altogether, in about a third it seems to make no difference, and for the rest their periods are lighter. The operation is much quicker and it is done as a day case. The post-operative recovery is much shorter (3 weeks) compared to hysterectomy, and overall there are fewer problems. It avoids the potential complications of hysterectomy, but satisfaction rates are similar in the long term. There is a small risk, about 1% of making a hole in the womb during the operation and you needing an emergency hysterectomy.

There are also some newer techniques that act in the same way, but can sometimes be done under local anaesthetic (Thermachoice balloon system, microwave endometrial ablation). These appear to be equally as successful.

Once the operation is performed, you are likely to have a discharge for 3–4 weeks. If you were to need HRT in the future you would have to take the hormone progesterone to protect the uterus lining, along with the estrogen that makes you feel well.

Thank you for telling me about the other treatments, but will either of them guarantee that I will have no more bleeding? I am fed up of having to carry sanitary towels everywhere and they are costing me a fortune. I don't want to have any other treatment. I want to have a hysterectomy.

No, the only thing that will guarantee that you will not have any further periods is a hysterectomy. However, do you know that hysterectomy is a major operation associated with risks of complications, such as excessive bleeding needing blood transfusion or further operations, injury to your bowel, bladder and the tube that carries urine from your kidney to your bladder. You could also suffer with anaesthetic complications and get chest and urinary tract infections. Because we handle the bowels during the operation they can stop working for a few days afterwards giving you severe stomachache. You are also at a higher risk of developing clots in your legs and lungs. After the operation you could get a wound infection and the wound could actually break down or later lead to a hernia. You could find afterwards that you develop bladder dysfunction and discomfort during sexual intercourse.

In fact, overall, the complication rate with abdominal hysterectomy is about 40% and with vaginal hysterectomy about 25%. The risk of dying from a hysterectomy is about 4–14 per 10 000 procedures.

If we were to perform a hysterectomy, the other thing we would need to consider is whether or not we should remove your ovaries. Removing your ovaries eliminates your risk of developing ovarian cancer, but would make you menopausal, and you would need to take HRT. The usual practice is to leave the ovaries at your age unless they are diseased, which is unlikely; but, in about one quarter of women the conserved ovaries fail to function within 2–5 years after the hysterectomy. The cause for this is unknown. It might be that failing ovarian function causes the heavy periods that lead to a subsequent hysterectomy, and they would have failed within a few years anyway. It is probable that disturbance of ovarian blood supply during and after a hysterectomy affects the ovaries leading to premature failure, or the ovaries fail to function in the absence of their target organ (the uterus). In this case you may require HRT despite the ovarian conservation. Removing the ovaries would make you menopausal instantaneously and expose you to the possibility of having long-term HRT.

I understand all these things and have thought long and hard about this. I am still keen to have a hysterectomy, despite its risks.

OK. When we perform a hysterectomy we remove the womb and the neck of the womb, so you will not need anymore smears, this is called a total hysterectomy. Some people ask for the neck of the womb to be left behind (subtotal hysterectomy). This is technically easy to do and has fewer complications such as bleeding and bladder dysfunction. It may also cause fewer disturbances to sexual function and help keep the top of the vagina supported, to reduce the chances of a prolapse. However, none of this is proven, and the disadvantages are that you may continue to have some menstrual spotting and will need cervical smears. (The chance of developing cervical stump carcinoma is under 1%).

There are three methods that we can use to perform a hysterectomy – these are through your stomach (abdominal), or your vagina or by a combination of both using keyhole surgery (laparoscopically assisted vaginal hysterectomy, LAVH). A total hysterectomy can be done each way, but, generally a sub-total cannot be done vaginally. When compared to an abdominal hysterectomy, the vaginal and keyhole operations are associated with fewer complications, a shorter hospital stay and quicker recovery afterwards.

I have not heard of this vaginal hysterectomy. Is it a new way or is it the suction method people talk about? What would you recommend for me.

No, it is not new. Vaginal hysterectomy was described in the days of Soranus of Ephesus (AD 120) and first performed by Langenbeck in 1813. Whereas abdominal hysterectomy is relatively new, Charles Clay in Manchester first performed it in 1844. I don't know where people get the idea that we use suction. Whichever way we do a hysterectomy we always cut the womb out.

In your case, as you have had three children born through your vagina, we ought to be able to perform a vaginal hysterectomy on you. I should be able to confirm that after I have examined you. Keyhole surgery is helpful in some cases as it increases the mobility of the womb by cutting the upper attachments through the camera in your tummy. The rest of the operation is then done vaginally. Basically, it converts a potential abdominal hysterectomy to a vaginal hyster-ectomy. Otherwise, you would have an abdominal hysterectomy with its increased risks of complications and longer recovery period. After you have had children your womb becomes more mobile. With a mobile womb a vaginal hysterectomy is usually possible and keyhole surgery does not provide much more advantage. Even if we do a vaginal or keyhole hysterectomy, there is always a possibility that we may have to open your tummy in case of any problem during the operation.

Thank you for explaining all that. I think I would prefer to have a vaginal hysterectomy, but what if I want my ovaries removed as well?

In most women, during hysterectomy the ovaries can be removed vaginally in 95–99% of cases. If the ovaries prove difficult to remove we could always remove them with the keyhole surgery.

Well, if possible I would like to have my ovaries left behind and it would be nice not to have a scar, so a vaginal hysterectomy sounds ideal. How long will I have to wait?

(The end of the consultation)

NB. In the examination there might be diagrams available to use as part of the consultation process. If not, feel free to draw some to help with your explanations.

Question E1

As part of the consultation you should have discussed a Mirena coil. Until recently these were only licensed in the UK as a method of contraception. As Mrs Thompson has been sterilized, clearly this is not a suitable indication.

Justify how you can prescribe a non-licensed treatment.

Your answer here ....

Question E2

You also mentioned endometrial ablation. If you were going to use a laser, which type of laser would you use for the ablation and why? How safe are the ablative methods and what are the other benefits in the treatment of menorrhagia?

Your answer here ....

CIRCUIT 2

Station F

It is 09.00 on a Sunday morning and you (the specialist registrar) walk on to the labour ward to start your 24-hour shift.

LABOUR WARD BOARD

Room	Name	Parity	Gestation	Comments	Midwife
HDU	Pinker	0+0	28	Twins. IVF pregnancy. Pre-eclampsia. MAGPIE Trial	Shelley and student
1	Chamberlin	0+1	42	Fully at 06.30. Pushing. Epidural.	Jane
2	Patel	0+3	15	Recurrent miscarriages For cervical suture Membranes bulging.	Nicky
3	Jeffcoate	3+2	39	Normal delivery 08.10. Placenta retained. Tear needs suturing.	Community MW (Adele)
4	Shaw	1+1	39	Previous CS. ARM 05.00. Slow progress	Caroline
5	Symmonds	5+0	40	Normal labour. 6cm at 08.30. Membranes intact. Previous shoulder dystocia	Sue
6	Blair	0+0	30	*Awaiting Dr.* ?SROM Occasional contractions	Monica
7	Bell	0+0	41	IOL for raised BP. 5cm at 06.00. Epidural ARM-Meconium. FBS at 08.45–pH 7.28	Karen
8	Fletcher	2+1	41	Spontaneous labour. 3cm at 06.00. Membranes intact.	Sue
9	Munro	1+1	22	Termination for Down's syndrome	Sally
10					

On the antenatal wards there are two women awaiting assessment for further prostaglandins. They are both post-mature primigravidae. There is another woman awaiting acceleration who is 39 weeks and it is 36 hours since her membranes ruptured.

On the gynaecological ward there are two problems. One lady had a vaginal hysterectomy yesterday afternoon and she has been bleeding quite heavily all night. The other is a 25-year-old girl admitted through casualty who appears to be having a miscarriage. Her pregnancy test is positive.

This is a unit delivering 3800 babies a year and you are on call with a consultant and associate specialist who are both at home – they normally telephone around 10 p.m. You have a junior SHO who is a competent career doctor with 14 months experience. The midwifery staff comprise Sue, the senior midwife, and two experienced midwives (Shelley and Jane) both competent at suturing, siting intravenous infusions and taking theatre cases. Of the other five midwives, only Caroline is trained for theatre. There is one community midwife, Adele, looking after a woman booked under the Domino scheme. There is one anaesthetic specialist registrar on duty with you.

Outline your management of the situation. Which of the antenatal women would you admit to room 10?

Your answer here ....

CIRCUIT 2

Question G1

You are called by your SHO to the casualty department to review Vanessa Powell, a 16-year-old girl who was found wandering in a local park. She is confused and disorientated in time and place but knows her name and address. She smelt of vomit and perhaps alcohol. She was unable to provide much history, but has given her parents' address. The casualty staff are currently trying to trace them. On examination she is dehydrated with a pulse of 96 beats per minute and a blood pressure of 180/105. They note she is unsteady on her feet and appears to have nystagmus. Abdominal examination reveals a pelvic mass equivalent to a uterus of 20 weeks' gestation and although they have not performed a pelvic examination, the casualty staff noticed that she appeared to be on a period. They have checked her urine and have sent bloods for a full blood count, basic biochemistry and a serum βhCG.

The results are:

Hb	10.2 g/dl
WCC	10.6×10^9
Plts	150×10^9
Na	125 mmol/l
K	2.8 mmol/l
U	10.2 mmol/l

Urine dip-stick:
Ketones	+++
Protein	+++
Glucose	negative
Blood	negative

Strongly positive serum pregnancy test

The staff have tried unsuccessfully to find a fetal heart beat and are confused about the diagnosis.

Outline your initial management and explain why you think this is necessary.

Your answer here ....

Question G2

You are unable to detect a fetal heart using a hand held Doppler and you request an urgent ultrasound scan. The scan findings show this:

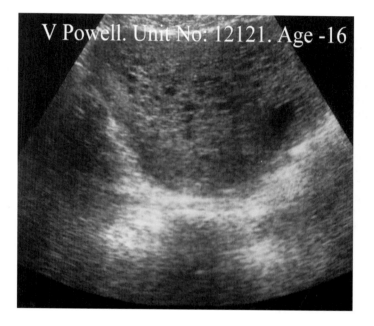

How would you describe this, what is your diagnosis and how will you confirm this?

Your answer here ... ...

Question G3

In view of the presumptive diagnosis, do you have any other concerns relating to Vanessa's condition? She still remains confused despite rehydration – what steps would you take next?

Your answer here ....

Question G4

Vanessa's condition remains unchanged, an MRI of her head is normal. The consultant feels that she has pre-eclampsia and needs to go to theatre as soon as the blood is cross-matched. Her parents have been found and come in to see you. They are Jehovah's witnesses, as is Vanessa. You ask them how she has been recently and they tell you she has been suffering with severe vomiting for the last 2 weeks. They are unaware of her pregnancy.

What would you tell them and what would you do next?

Your answer here ....

Question G5

Vanessa is taken to theatre and has an uneventful uterine evacuation. Her blood pressure settles over the next few days and her consciousness level improves. She is discharged home on day 3 and you see her the following week for review. Her histology reveals a complete mole.

What do you know about the types and aetiology of molar pregnancies? Explain the subsequent management to her and her parents.

Your answer here ....

CIRCUIT 2

Question H1

Janice Gregory, a 28-year-old secretary of mixed race referred herself to the antenatal clinic when 32 weeks pregnant, saying that she had not felt the baby move during the last 24 hours.

She is married and lives with her husband, a teacher who has gone to work. This is her first pregnancy. The pregnancy was planned and she booked for antenatal care at 10 weeks. She was in good general health, did not smoke, drank no alcohol and was not on any medications. She underwent routine booking blood tests. She was found to have a rhesus negative blood group and the antibody screen was negative. All other results were reported as normal. Her dating ultrasound scan agreed with her dates, when calculated from her last menstrual period. Shared care was arranged. An anomaly scan at 19 weeks was reported as normal. The course of her pregnancy was uncomplicated, except for an episode of post-coital bleeding at 30 weeks when she had attended the casualty department and been reassured.

She was last seen in the antenatal clinic at 28 weeks. Maternal observations and urinanalysis were normal. The symphysis-fundal height was 29 cm. She was well. The baby was active, lying longitudinally with a breech presentation. The fetal heartbeat was audible.

On review in the antenatal clinic today the woman appears concerned but well. There is no obvious cause for absent fetal movements. There is no vaginal discharge or bleeding. Her blood pressure is normal (130/80 mmHg) and urine clear. The symphysis-fundal height was 33 cm, the lie longitudinal and the presentation remains a breech.

How would you make a conclusive diagnosis of fetal death?

Your answer here ....

Question H2

An ultrasound scan was performed, these were the results:

Faith Hospital Department of Radiology

Name: **Janice Gregory**
Age: **28**
Unit number: **34576**

The uterus contains a single fetus, presenting as a footling breech. The heart is seen but there is no fetal heart beat or movements present. The gross anatomy appears normal. The bladder is empty and Spalding's sign is positive. Liquor is slightly reduced, maximum pool – 3 cm. The placenta is fundal.

HC   285 mm
AC   245 mm
FL   55 mm

Radiologist: **Carol Claytons, / Andrea Linch**

The 19-week scan had measured the head circumference (HC) as 152 mm and the abdominal circumference (AC) as 124 mm.

What would you tell Janice and what action would you take at this stage?

What management options are available?

Your answer here ....

Your answer here (cont.) ....

Question H3

What are the advantages and disadvantages of expectant management?

What options are available for the induction of labour?

Your answer here ....

Question H4

At Janice's request, the labour was induced with mifepristone the next morning. 36 hours later and following a favourable vaginal examination she was prescribed vaginal prostaglandins. An ARM was performed and an intravenous syntocinon infusion commenced the subsequent day. The labour was uneventful, culminating in the delivery of a normal looking male fetus with no signs of life. Macroscopically it was a normal looking placenta. The amniotic fluid was slightly meconium stained, and there was minimal maceration of the fetus. The estimated blood loss was 400 ml.

What findings at birth could help in establishing the cause of the death?

Which fetal and maternal investigations would you recommend?

Your answer here ....

Question H5

The early post-partum period was uncomplicated. All the samples for further evaluation were taken and the investigations arranged. On the second day post-partum Janice wanted to go home. What would you do before allowing her home?

Your answer here ....

CIRCUIT 2

Question 11

It is 13.00 on Friday afternoon and you are due to start operating in the Day Care Unit at 14.00. It is always a busy list and you insist on seeing your pre-operative patients first, even though they have been seen in a pre-operative clinic. Your consultant never attends and you are assisted by a nurse practitioner when necessary. Today on the list you have a cone biopsy, two laparoscopic sterilizations, a diagnostic laparoscopy for deep dyspareunia, two laparoscopies for infertility and two hysteroscopies for irregular and post-menopausal bleeding.

The last patient you see is Mrs Nicky Dean, who is fourth on the list. She is due to have a laparoscopy to investigate the cause of her deep dyspareunia. She has developed the problem over the last 18 months since her caesarean section. She also notices pain on defecation (dyschezia) and pelvic pain when she has her periods. A provisional diagnosis of endometriosis has been made and she is having her laparoscopy to confirm this. She was listed for the operation 8 months ago.

In the 5 minutes before the list starts, what would you say to Mrs Dean?

Your answer here ....

Question 12

You perform your laparoscopy and insert the Veress needle at the third attempt, because she is overweight. The intra-abdominal pressure registers −2 mmHg and you start to insufflate the abdomen. After you have put 2.5 l of carbon dioxide into the abdomen you insert your trochar. On inserting the laparoscope you can see extensive adhesions between the omentum and anterior abdominal wall, possibly due to her previous section. The adhesions are obscuring your view of the uterus and the left adnexum. You try and move the laparoscope forwards and to the right of these adhesions to visualise the uterus. As you move the laparoscope the adhesions seem to follow you and the laparoscope seems to 'snag'. In fact it is difficult to move the laparoscope from side to side. You wander why this has happened and looking back to the left-hand side you see what you think is fecal material loose in the abdominal cavity.

What are your immediate thoughts, and what will you initially do to try and confirm your findings?

Your answer here ....

Question 13

You insert a second trochar suprapubically and looking up to the umbilicus see that the sigmoid colon is adherent to the umbilicus and your first trochar has gone straight through it.

Your consultant is not on call and not traceable. What are your next steps?

Your answer here ....

Question 14

You finally trace a general surgeon who is on call but is currently finishing a thyroidectomy. She informs you that she will be about half an hour, has limited laparoscopic skills and that your patient will require a laparotomy to repair the bowel damage. She suggests you make a start.

How would you proceed?

Your answer here ....

Question 15

The surgeon arrives and confirms that the sigmoid colon was adherent to the umbilicus. She initially mobilized this fully and then inspected the rest of the large and small bowel to look for other injuries. She repaired the exit wound with Vicryl on the posterior surface of the sigmoid, and then decided to perform a loop colostomy using the entry wound as the stoma. Mrs Dean makes an excellent post-operative recovery and is discharged after a week. Four months later she has her stoma successfully reversed. A year later a copy of the following letter arrives.

BANNISTERS SOLICITORS

Dear Sirs
Re: Mrs Nicola Dean
     32, Hartley Street, London

We are representing Mrs Nicola Dean who on the afternoon of Friday 13th March attended your day case unit for a routine laparoscopy to investigate the cause of her pain. During the operation her bowel was damaged in two separate places. A specialist bowel surgeon then needed to be called to repair the damage.

Our client alleges negligence during the course of the operation, which resulted in the necessity of a temporary stoma. This has scarred her both mentally and physically. Her body image has changed, she no longer wishes to reveal any part of her abdomen which makes swimming with her son and holidays impossible. She also suffered with depression following the operation and has regular abdominal pains.

Please find enclosed Protocol ProForma with supporting documentation.

Yours faithfully
BANNISTERS

Please comment on the allegations.

Your answer here ....

CIRCUIT 2

Question J1

Janet Hooper is a 28-year-old caucasian woman who is booking in the antenatal clinic of her district general hospital, when 14 weeks pregnant in her second pregnancy, following a normal scan. Her first pregnancy had culminated in an emergency lower segment caesarean section 3 years previously for slow progress in the first stage of labour. Her newborn son weighed 3.5 kg and her recovery after the operation was uncomplicated. There is no further information available about her previous pregnancy and delivery, because she had recently moved house.

She tells you that she had a very unpleasant experience with her first delivery and is worried about the mode of delivery this time. Otherwise, her obstetric and gynaecological history is uncomplicated. She is in good general health. The course of the current pregnancy until now has been uneventful. She is keen to avoid a further caesarean delivery if possible, and certainly does not want to go through a similar experience to last time.

How would you counsel her regarding the mode of delivery in this pregnancy?

Your answer here ....

Question J2

What methods of investigation are currently available for assessing the chances of vaginal delivery for this woman and what is their value?

Your answer here ....

Question J3

Janet opts for a trial of labour, even at this early stage of her pregnancy, but wishes to review the situation at 36 weeks as you suggest. She has her triple test and is due to see you after her normality scan at 20 weeks.

The triple test comes back as normal, but the AFP is raised. What would you advise?

Your answer here ....

Question J4

She has a detailed ultrasound scan the following day when 18 weeks pregnant. The scan demonstrates a large midline abdominal wall defect. This is incorporating the umbilicus, and the bowel is seen to be herniating through the anterior abdominal wall. You have kindly offered to see her on the antenatal day unit for follow up.

What would be your explanation and recommendations now?

Your answer here ....

Question J5

The pregnancy progresses without complications. She is seen in antenatal clinic at 37 weeks. A scan last week confirmed a well-grown fetus, presenting cephalically, a posterior placenta and normal liquor volume.

She wants to further discuss details of the labour and delivery.

Your answer here ....

CIRCUIT 2

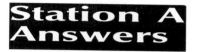

Answer A1

By definition, the menopause means the last menstrual period. It can only be accurately diagnosed retrospectively 1 year after this period. This lady is therefore peri-menopausal. She is symptomatic with predominantly vasomotor symptoms, but her gonadotrophins and estradiol levels do not confirm complete ovarian failure. Her TSH is mildly elevated (normal <6) and her thyroxine level is low (normal >70) indicating a degree of hypothyroidism which may be contributing to her symptomatology (weight gain, depression, loss of libido, oligomenorrhoea and hypertension).

I would examine her neck for a goitre and check her thyroid auto-antibodies. Thus, in the first instance I would wish to commence her on thyroxine (initially 50 μg/day) increasing gradually as required. I would then refer her to an endocrinologist and arrange a review in 3 months time.

I would also advise her to use a method of contraception. Not only is she at risk of pregnancy because she is perimenopausal, but correcting her thyroid function may cause her periods to resume. (Theoretically she could be pregnant at present and so you may wish to consider performing a pregnancy test.)

Answer A2

This woman still has a uterus, so in order to minimize the risk of endometrial carcinoma she will require a combined preparation containing both oestrogen and progestogen. It is now 10 months since her last period, so it would be inappropriate to commence a continuous combined preparation with its associated irregular bleeding patterns.

I would discuss the various ways of administering HRT with the woman – orally, transdermally, percutaneously, nasally or as implants, and would explain that the different preparations are all equally as effective. If she had no strong feelings about the mode of administration, I would commence her on a low dose oral preparation because they are much more cost effective than other methods. I would explain that she could take estrogen tablets on a daily basis with progestogen added in for the last 2 weeks of each month (Climagest, Cyclo-progynova, Elleste Duet, Femoston, Nuvelle, Premique Cycle, Prempak-C, Trisequens) or every 3 months (Tridestra). If she was not keen on taking multiple tablets, Prempak-C would not be advisable because during the second half of the cycle she would need to take two separate tablets. All of the other preparations involve only a single tablet.

I would also explain that the estrogen could be delivered via a patch, aerosol, implant or cream and pessary. If she chose any of these she would still require oral progestogens during the second half of each cycle. If she did not wish to take any tablets, she could be prescribed a combined patch (Estracombi, Evorel Sequi, Nuvelle TS). The advantages of patches are that they provide more constant hormone levels and only need to be changed every 3–4 days, but may cause local skin reactions, sometimes adhere poorly and are a much more expensive form of currently available preparations.

She could have an estradiol implant inserted under local anaesthetic. This provides a much more stable and lower dose of serum estradiol, but may be associated with tachyphylaxis. As lack of libido is a problem, this could be a treatment option because testosterone can be added at the same time. She would need to take progestogen tablets for the last 2 weeks of every month to stimulate a withdrawal bleed.

The only other alternative way to deliver the protective benefits of progestogens is by using the levonorgestrel-releasing intrauterine system (Mirena). This could be inserted and she could be prescribed estrogen patches, gels, tablets or implants with this. This would be suitable if she was concerned about her risk of pregnancy with condoms or her periods had been heavy in the past.

As vasomotor symptoms are one of her predominant symptoms I do not feel that a selective oestrogen receptor modulator (SERM) like Evista or bone regulators would be appropriate forms of treatment for her. Thus, if she had no preference on administration routes I would commence her on an oral preparation such as 1 mg ElleStearet, which is the cheapest HRT available at present, and contains a low dose of estradiol, the most physiological form of estrogen (rather than conjugated estrogens). It also contains norethisterone an androgenic progesterone which may help with her libido.

Answer A3

This problem of irregular bleeding occurs in 16.8–19.3% of cycles in women using cyclical HRT regimes. The commonest pattern is withdrawal bleeding or spotting (77–81.3%) lasting for 6.5–7 days and 3.4–3.5 days, respectively, and some women (16.1–18.8%) experience amenorrhoea.

There are many possible causes of bleeding in a woman on cyclical HRT, some physiological, some pathological. They include poor compliance (which is the most likely cause), poor absorption of the medication in the gastro-intestinal tract (associated with broad-spectrum antibiotics) and failure to synchronize the HRT with the endogenous cycle of the woman. Other causes include gynaecological pathology (vaginal, cervical, endometrial), drug-related effects (previous use of estradiol implants, concomitant administration of liver enzyme inducers or anticoagulants), and clotting defects.

The woman needs to be examined and after ruling out vaginal and cervical causes, endometrial pathology needs to be excluded by performing an endometrial biopsy. This can be combined with either hysteroscopy (preferably as an outpatient) or a transvaginal ultrasound scan. The transvaginal scan can be combined with saline endometrial perfusion if submucous fibroids or polyps are suspected.

Answer A4

I would explain to her that the results from the laboratory have revealed that the lining of her uterus is thickened. I would reassure her that there is little to worry about. Hyperplasia without atypical cells is rarely associated with the development of endometrial carcinoma (under 1%), but we should keep this under surveillance.

The recurrence of the vasomotor symptoms suggests that the dose of estradiol may be insufficient and it might be helpful to increase the dose to 2 mg of estradiol daily.

The progestogenic side effects are physical and are probably related to the fact that norethisterone is an androgenic progestogen. A less androgenic form could be tried (dydrogesterone, medroxyprogesterone acetate) or the duration of administration lowered. The disadvantage of shortening the duration of progestogen exposure is that it will increase the risks of hyperplasia (which she already has). Further management options could include inserting a Mirena coil or trying a vaginal progesterone gel, adding in a weak diuretic for the last week of the cycle (to help with the fluid retention symptoms). Sometimes, increasing the dose of progestogen or adding an androgen may help. Although it might cause her to have irregular bleeds, she could try Tibolone as a different oral therapeutic option. An alternative approach would be to offer her a hysterectomy (with or without bilateral salpingo-oophorectomy) with subsequent estrogen-only HRT.

Answer A5

In view of the fact that she has recurrent vaginal bleeds in the presence of endometrial hyperplasia, the minimum she would require is a hysteroscopy and further endometrial sampling. I would also counsel her about a hysterectomy, and examine her to see if a vaginal hysterectomy is possible because of its shorter recovery time.

Answer A6

She can start the HRT immediately. If there was some residual function in her ovaries her estradiol levels would be falling in the first 24 hours postoperatively. I would advise a 2 mg estradiol tablet in the first instance, but would obviously discuss the options of implants and patches.

There are two main risks associated with the use of HRT: deep vein thrombosis (DVT) and breast cancer. The risk of a DVT is one extra case per year for every 5000 patients, but this is increased in the presence of other risk factors such as personal and family history and obesity. The risk of breast cancer increases in relation to duration of use. It increases after 5 years of use from 45/1000 to 47/

1000 (not statistically significant); after 10 years of use it increases to 51/1000 and after 20 years of use to 57/1000. However, the breast cancers associated with HRT users tend to be more localized, less advanced at the time of diagnosis and have a better prognosis. Following the discontinuation of the HRT the risk reduces and almost disappears after 5 years. On balance, the benefits from HRT predominate when used for up to 10 years, and this should be reinforced.

Further reading

Archer DF, Pickar JH, Bottiglioni F (1994) Menopause Study Group. Bleeding patterns in women taking continuous combined or sequential regimes of conjugated oestrogens with medroxyprogesterone acetate. *Obstet. Gynecol.* **83**: 686–692.

Barlow D (1997) Who understands the menopause? *Br. J. Obstet. Gynaecol.* **107**: 879–880.

(1996) Hormone replacement therapy. *Drug Therapeut. Bull.* **34**: 81–84.

(1996) Menopausal disorders. *Monthly Index of Medical Specialities,* June: 342–361.

Rogerson L, Jones S (1998) The investigation of women with post-menopausal bleeding. PACE Review No. 98/07. Royal College of Obstetricians and Gynaecologists, London.

Rosenberg S, Kroll M, Vandromme J (1996) Decision factors influencing hormone replacement therapy. *Br. J. Obstet. Gynaecol.* **103** (Suppl.): 92–98.

Slade R *et al.* Hormone replacement therapy. *Key Topics in Obstetrics and Gynaecology*, p. 50. BIOS Scientific Publishers Ltd, Oxford.

Spencer CP, Cooper AJ, Whitehead MI (1997) Management of abnormal bleeding in women receiving hormone replacement therapy. *Br. Med. J.* **315**: 37–42.

Studd J (1998) The management of the menopause. *Annual Review 1998*. Parthenon Publishing, Lancashire.

Sturdee DW (1997) Newer HRT regimens. *Br. J. Obstet. Gynaecol.* **104**: 1109–1115.

Wise J (1997) Hormone replacement therapy increases risk of breast cancer. *Br. Med. J.* **315**: 969.

CIRCUIT 2

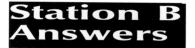

Answer B1

I would tell the midwife to contact the on-call SHO and anaesthetist at once, with instructions to obtain venous access. I would also ask her to inform the porters that they will be needed for urgent samples and notify the laboratories. I would then go to the labour ward immediately to assess the woman.

After ensuring basic life support (ABC), I would take a brief history of the woman (either from her or the attending relatives or midwife) *whilst assessing her clinical condition and beginning treatment simultaneously.*

I would ask a few general questions (this might be to the patient, her partner or the midwife, as appropriate), initially about her age, parity, previous deliveries (caesarean sections, post-partum haemorrhages), this pregnancy (pregnancy induced hypertension), its duration, and the type of labour (spontaneous or induced). I would also ask about co-existing medical conditions, concomitant medications and religion (Jehovah's Witness).

I would then ask more specific questions relating to the labour. I would enquire as to the length of the second and third stages and the weight of the baby, the type of analgesia used during labour, the use of Syntometrine, whether or not the placenta had been expelled and if it was complete. I would ascertain if an episiotomy was performed or perineal tear had occurred, and the amount of blood loss since delivery (and her most recent haemoglobin).

While doing this, I would ask either the SHO or anaesthetist to site two intravenous lines with 14 gauge cannulas and to withdraw blood to send urgently for a full blood count, urea and electrolytes, blood group and cross-match (4–6 units depending on the blood loss) and the coagulation profile. I would commence a rapid infusion of crystalloids (utilizing pressure cuffs) and would ask someone to document the times and any drugs used. I would ask a midwife to prepare 500 ml of normal saline containing 40 IU of syntocinon to run at 125 ml (10 IU) per hour.

I would check her level of consciousness, pulse rate, blood pressure and presence of pallor to assess the general condition of the woman. I would then begin to look for the cause of the bleeding. I would perform a quick abdominal examination to check the height of the uterus, whether it is contracted or not, and for any tenderness (for example, scar rupture in presence of uterine scar). During the abdominal examination I would massage the uterus noting whether it contracts well. I would check for signs of placental separation (if it has not been expelled) and perform a quick vaginal assessment looking for the presence of any genital tract tears or trauma (labial, perineal, vaginal or cervical) and the presence of any active bleeding.

It is always worth observing the blood to see if it has clotted. If the estimated blood loss is more than 1000 ml I would inform the on-call obstetric consultant and haematologist and ask for group specific un-crossmatched blood.

If the bleeding stops without any evidence of a definite cause and the woman remains stable, I would document the estimated blood loss, continue the intravenous syntocinon infusion, monitor her general condition and check her haemoglobin level. The commonest cause of post-partum haemorrhage is uterine atony, hence the decision for the early use of intravenous syntocinon. If the uterus is well contracted, and prior to giving further drugs to treat this, the other causes of haemorrhage need to be eliminated.

If the placenta were retained with continued bleeding, I would arrange for an urgent manual removal in theatre, under a general anaesthetic, considering the possibility of a morbidly adherent placenta. I would request a general anaesthetic in case we needed to undertake any other major procedures and regional anaesthesia would further compromise her blood pressure. After cleaning and draping the patient, and catheterizing her, I would insert my right hand into her vagina with my fingers together almost at a point. If the cervix were closed I would gradually open my fingers to dilate the cervix. If halothane were available I would discuss its use with the anaesthetist. Once my hand was in the uterus, I would place my left hand over the fundus of the uterus (abdominally). I would then identify the plane of cleavage between the placenta and the uterus and try to separate them with my fingertips, removing the placenta as a whole (if possible). I would examine the cavity to ensure that it was empty and check the cervix for any lacerations with sponge forceps. Finally, I would suture any tears or an episiotomy. During the operation I would continue the syntocinon infusion and ask for a dose of intravenous antibiotics. The syntocinon infusion should be continued for the next 4 hours after the manual removal to keep the uterus contracted.

If the woman is severely shocked, to a greater degree than would be expected given her blood loss, the possibility of uterine inversion must be considered. The placenta may be adherent (50%) and a bluish-grey mass might be seen extruding from the perineum. If this is the case, prompt action is essential. The uterus needs to be reinstated as quickly as possible, either digitally or by utilizing hydrostatic pressure. I would grasp the fundus of the uterus with my right hand, with the fingers directed towards the posterior fornix and forcefully lift the uterus out of the pelvis by pushing my forearm up the vagina. If she were bradycardic she would also require atropine and IV fluids, and once the uterus has everted an syntocinon infusion should be commenced.

If the placenta has been removed and the uterus is well contracted, the bleeding may be perineal, vaginal or cervical in origin. An adequate examination (often in theatre) may be necessary to identify the bleeding points and suture them appropriately. An episiotomy should be repaired in layers with an absorbable synthetic polyglycolic acid (Vicryl or Dexon). The skin should be closed with a subcuticular suture. Swabs and needles require checking and vaginal and rectal examinations performed.

[NB. You could be given a model of a perineum with a tear or episiotomy and asked to suture it. Be able to justify your technique.]

If the bleeding is excessive, appears to be of uterine origin and there is no other obvious cause, a uterine rupture should be suspected. This can occur spontaneously, but is more common with previous uterine scars. An examination under anaesthesia may reveal the defect and an urgent laparotomy with repair is required.

Rarely, coagulopathies may present this way, hence the need to check platelet levels and coagulation times. The correct management is to treat the cause.

If the bleeding is due to an atonic uterus, I would start to compress and elevate the uterus bimanually. Elevation of the uterus stretches the uterine artery thereby reducing the blood loss. The other method to reduce blood loss is to compress the aorta against the sacral promontory. If it has not already been prescribed, I would give one dose of syntometrine intravenously. If the bleeding still continues after 5 minutes, I would ask the SHO to give 250 μg of carboprost intramyometrially while continuing bimanual compression and elevation of the uterus. If carboprost is not available, one or two 1 mg gemeprost pessaries can be inserted inside the uterine cavity.

Answer B2

The situation is now becoming desperate. By definition this is a massive primary post-partum haemorrhage (PPH) (blood loss in excess of 1000 ml). With this amount of bleeding the blood loss estimate should be doubled, and the fact that the blood is no longer clotting suggests a coagulopathy. It is imperative to involve the consultant haematologist on call and to repeat all of her blood tests. Group-specific blood is required immediately, and if this is not available O-negative blood should be given. The SHO should continue to try and contact the consultant on call, and should ask the hospital switchboard to contact the other consultants who work in the unit.

The cause of the bleeding is an atonic uterus and simple pharmacological methods have failed. If she was still conscious I would discuss the situation with the patient and inform her that the situation was grave and that she required transfer to theatre. I would consent her for a laparotomy and proceed and explain that she might end up with a hysterectomy. I would also keep her partner aware of the situation.

I would discuss the situation with the anaesthetist and arrange to take her to theatre. Once she is asleep, in the first instance I would try to tamponade the uterus by inserting a Sengstaken-Blakemore tube or a Foley's catheter with large bulb inside the uterus and inflate it with 300 ml of saline. I would continue the syntocinon infusion during this time, and ask for an intravenous injection of

100 mg Tranexamic acid. If this was successful in managing the bleeding the tube/catheter should be left for 24 hours, then deflated slowly by about 20 ml per hour. Another alternative is to pack the uterus with 10 cm wide gauze (5 m in length) for 24 hours. (Beware of concealed bleeding despite these measures.)

The only other conservative method to control the bleeding is radiographic embolization of both the internal iliac arteries, but this requires a radiologist expert in performing angiography.

Answer B3

The woman needs a laparotomy to save her life. She has now developed disseminated intravascular coagulopathy and any surgical insult will result in further bleeding. It is imperative that she receives platelets and continues to receive blood.

I would perform a laparotomy through a midline incision, as this is generally thought to be less vascular, and just in case there is a rare cause for her bleeding or associated pathology. Before commencing with a sub-total hysterectomy, I would initially ligate the uterine arteries and veins bilaterally. To do this I would grasp the round ligament and incise it to divide the leaves of the broad ligament, I would separate them with my fingers and continue this blunt dissection to the pelvic side walls to identify the ureters. I would then find the uterine vessels and ligate them. If this did not work I would continue to ligate the infundibulopelvic vessels and perform a sub-total hysterectomy. The final procedure would be ligation of the internal iliac arteries if all else fails and the coagulopathy is corrected.

Prior to closing I would insert a drain and would wait for the arrival of the consultant to ensure she is happy with haemostasis.

Answer B4

Once the operation was over I would fully explain the operation to the relatives of the woman. I would write my notes up fully and retrospectively and ensure the woman was monitored in a high dependency area.

I would then complete a critical incident form. Not only was the massive haemorrhage a critical incident, but perhaps of more importance was the unavailability of the consultant on call.

Answer B5

Yes, the B-Lynch technique can be used effectively to treat bleeding in this case.

A number 1 Vicryl suture is passed from the outside inwards, through the lower flap of the opened lower segment about 3 cm below the cut margin, and is taken out from the inside outwards, through the upper flap of the lower segment about 4 cm above the cut margin. The suture is then passed over the top of the fundus of the uterus and is inserted from the outside inwards, through the posterior wall about 4 cm above the cut margin on the anterior wall. It is continued laterally for about 3 cm inside the uterus and is passed from the inside outwards, again through the posterior uterine wall about 4 cm above the cut margin on the anterior wall. It is then continued over the top of the fundus in a reverse direction to go through the upper and lower flaps of the incision anteriorly at the same level as on the other side. The two ends of the suture are tied over the lower flap of the cut lower segment. This technique is described as being quite effective in stopping bleeding from the uterus following caesarean section and can save the uterus in most cases.

Further reading

B-Lynch C, Coker A, Lawal AH, Abu J, Cowen MJ (1997) The B-Lynch surgical technique for the control of massive postpartum haemorrhage: an alternative to hysterectomy? Five cases reported. *Br. J. Obstet. Gynaecol.* **104**: 372–375.

Drife J (1997) Management of primary post partum haemorrhage. *Br. J. Obstet. Gynaecol.* **104**: 275–277.

Royal College of Obstetricians and Gynaecologists (2000) Methods and materials used in perineal repair. RCOG Guideline No. 23. Royal College of Obstetricians and Gynaecologists, London

Slade R et al. (1998) Post-partum haemorrhage. Key Topics in Obstetrics and Gynaecology, pp. 266–269. BIOS Scientific Publishers Ltd, Oxford.

CIRCUIT 2

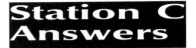

LAST CHANCE NHS TRUST
CONSENT FORM FOR FEMALE STERILIZATION

Patient's Surname   Other Names

Unit Number   Date of Birth

Instructions to the Doctor (This part to be completed by a suitably qualified doctor)

Type of operation: Sterilization

I confirm that I have explained the procedure, associated risks (listed below), and any anaesthetic (general/regional) required, to the patient in terms that in my judgement are suited to her understanding.

Signature   Date

Name of doctor   Grade

Instructions to the Patient

1 Please read this form very carefully.
2 If there is anything that you don't understand about the explanation, or if you want more information, you should ask the doctor.
3 Please check that all the information on the form is correct. If it is, and you understand the explanation, then sign and initial the form where indicated.

Please note:
The doctor is here to help you. He or she will explain the proposed procedure, which you are entitled to refuse. You can ask any questions and seek further information.

You may ask for a relative, or friend, or a nurse to be present.

Training doctors and other health professionals is essential to the continuation of the health service and improving the quality of care. Your treatment may provide an important opportunity for such training, where necessary under the careful supervision of a senior doctor. *You may, however, decline to be involved in the formal training of medical and other students without this adversely affecting your care and treatment.*

NAME . . . .   UNIT NUMBER . . . .

I am the patient.

I agree to have this operation, which has been explained to me by the doctor named above.

I agree to have the type of anaesthetic that I have been told about, but understand that the type of anaesthetic used is decided by the anaesthetist.

I understand that the operation might not be done by the doctor who has been treating me up until now, and that doctors in training might be involved.

Please initial

I understand that:

- the aim of the operation is to stop me having children;   ———
- it might not be possible to reverse the effects of the operation, and I may have to pay for this privately;   ———
- sterilization can sometimes fail, and that there is a very small chance that I may become fertile again after some time;   ———
- if I do become pregnant there is more chance that it will be outside my uterus (an ectopic pregnancy);   ———
- if I was pregnant at the moment the operation should not affect it;   ———
- there are significant risks of a laparotomy;   ———
- it might affect my periods;   ———
- I should take other precautions until my next period;   ———
- vasectomy is as effective but safer.   ———

I also understand that any procedure in addition to the investigation or treatment described on this form will only be carried out if it is necessary and in my best interests and can be justified for medical reasons.

I have told the doctor about the procedures listed below I would not wish to be carried out straightaway without my having the opportunity to consider them first.

Signature

Answer C1

Consent implies permission from the patient to undergo an examination, investigation or operation.

Every competent adult has the right to give or withhold his or her consent. In fact, patient autonomy is the guiding principle of medical law. There is no law of proxy in English law, so no adult can give consent on behalf of another adult. Only the patient can give consent. The principle of self-determination would in most circumstances prevail even above the sanctity of life. To perform even an examination without consent can lead to dire consequences (an action for damages, criminal proceedings, and even professional misconduct). By the law of trespass, a doctor who proceeds to act in the absence of consent would be liable for trespass, assault or battery, without the need for proof. By the law of negligence, there is an obligation to provide information identifying risks. In common law a patient can only be treated when he/she gives consent.

In law, a competent adult is defined as a person who has reached 18 years of age and has the capacity to make treatment decisions on his own behalf. Capacity is implied if the patient can comprehend and retain the treatment information, believe that information and weigh it in the balance to arrive at a choice. If an adult is incompetent then in law no other adult can take responsibility for him or her. This might arise through an unconscious state and mental incapacity. In this case doctors must act in the best interests of their patients, and abide by any ascertainable past wishes (living wills), and provide a standard of care laid down in Bolam (in accordance with a reasonable body of relevant professional opinion).

Parents give consent for the treatment of their child. The legal age of consent for medical or surgical treatment is 16 years or over (Section 8 of the Family Law Reform Act 1969); however, a competent child (16–18 years old) cannot always veto treatment that parents have authorized. The absence of parents does not preclude treatment, but consent still needs to be obtained from 'loco parentis' (another relative or guardian). If a child is in care, the local authority acquires parental control (Children's Act, 1989).

The right of children under the age of 16 to give consent is encompassed under the Gillick judgement (1985). They can only give consent to treatment if they understand its nature, purpose and hazards.

The Clinical Negligence Scheme for Trusts operated by the NHS Litigation Authority states 'a person capable of performing the procedure' should take the consent. Ideally, it is the responsibility of the person providing treatment (doctor, nurse or dentist) or undertaking an investigation, to discuss it with the patient and obtain consent, as they have a comprehensive understanding of the procedure or treatment, how it is carried out, and the risks involved. If this is not possible, it should be someone who is suitably trained and qualified and with sufficient knowledge and understanding of the procedure to discuss fully the details and associated risks, and acts in accordance with the guidance of the General Medical Council.

Answer C2

Successful relationships between doctors and patients depend on trust and not everything that we do requires written consent. Consent is implied for most examinations when the patient undresses, similarly by offering their arm for venepuncture. Expressed consent is either oral or written and is necessary prior to any procedure that carries a risk. If oral consent has been obtained initially, it is advisable to gain written consent later or at the very least to document in the notes why written consent was not obtained.

It is not essential to take written consent for most procedures. It must be obtained for some treatments covered by statutory requirements (e.g. some fertility treatments licensed by the Human Fertilisation and Embryo Authority).

It is important to ensure that the patient has understood and agreed to undergo the procedure proposed and to keep a written record of the nature of information provided, specific requests by the patient and details of the scope of the consent given. Written consent should be taken where:

- the procedure is complex and associated with significant potential risks and/or side effects;

- the primary purpose of the procedure is not to provide clinical care;

- there is the possibility of significant consequences for the patient's employment, personal or social life;

- the procedure is part of a research.

Answer C3

Under certain circumstances a patient can be treated without informed consent. In an emergency, where consent cannot be obtained, medical treatment may be provided as long as the treatment is limited to what is immediately necessary to save a life or to avoid significant deterioration in the patient's health. Any valid advance refusal (which is known at that time) must be respected. Once the patient is sufficiently recovered to understand, the treatment and its reason should be explained to him/her.

In mentally incapacitated patients, treatment judged to be in their best interests may be carried out, provided they comply. However, if they do not comply, they may be compulsorily treated for any mental disorder only within the safeguards laid down by the Mental Health Act 1983. They may also be treated for any physical disorder arising from that mental disorder, in line with the guidance in the Code of Practice of the Mental Health Commission. A court's approval should be sought for any non-therapeutic or controversial treatments that are not directed at a mental disorder.

While treating a patient who has lost capacity to consent to treatment, or refuses treatment through onset, or progress of a mental disorder or other disability, an advance statement (living wills or advance directives) indicating preferences must be respected. This is provided that the decision in the advance statement is clearly applicable to the present circumstances, and there is no reason to believe that the patient has changed his or her mind. In the absence of an advance statement, the patient's known wishes should be considered.

NB. In Scotland, a 'tutor-dative' with appropriate authority may make medical decisions on behalf of a mentally incapacitated patient. Also, persons with parental responsibility cannot authorise procedures a competent child has refused. Legal advice may be helpful in such cases.

Answer C4

The options are decided following the 'best interests' principle that takes into account the following:

- clinically indicated options for treatment and investigation;

- the patient's previously expressed preferences (advance statement);

- knowledge of the patient's background (e.g. cultural, religious, employment);

- views about the patient's preferences given by a third party (e.g. partner, family, tutor-dative in Scotland, or a person with parental responsibility);

- the option that is least restrictive for patient's future choices.

It is also important to seek the views of senior colleagues, consider talking to your defence union or ascertaining the views of the Royal College.

Answer C5

A signed consent form is not sufficient evidence that a patient has given, or still gives, informed consent to the proposed treatment in all its aspects. Therefore, I would review the consent by checking that she still needs the operation and she is still happy to have it. I would reiterate the operation and potential risks, highlighting any potentially relevant information that might have appeared in the last 2 months, and discuss alternative treatment options. I would not re-consent her unless things had changed.

Further reading

GMC *Seeking patients' consent: the ethical considerations.* General Medical Council, London.
MDU *Consent to treatment.* The Medical Defence Union, London.

CIRCUIT 2

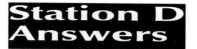
Station D Answers

Answer D1

First, I would ask the midwife to reassure Mrs Park. I would point out that she may well have been affected as a child without knowing it. I would inform her that chickenpox is a very common childhood illness, and over three-quarters of the adult population are immune. Reassuringly, although contact is common in pregnancy, infection is rare (about 1 in 2000 pregnancies).

Her friend's son would have been infectious when she saw him, because the disease is infectious for 2 days before the rash appears and remains so until the vesicles crust over. We would need to confirm that it actually is chickenpox that the boy is suffering from and to ascertain details of her contact with him because the virus is passed both by direct contact and airborne transmission. The risk of an infection is also significant if the contact with an infected person was indoors for more than 1 hour, or face-to-face for 5 minutes.

The prodromal illness may include a headache, but occurs 2–3 weeks after initial exposure. Therefore, her headache is likely to be due to anxiety or some other cause rather than chickenpox developing.

We need to establish whether or not Mrs Park is immune to the Varicella zoster virus, so I would ask the midwife to take a serum sample with the booking bloods. The virology laboratory can then check for the Varicella zoster immunoglobulin G (IgG) in the serum.

I would suggest that if Mrs Park remained anxious she could come to the next antenatal clinic to discuss the situation and for us to scan her to confirm fetal viability and her dates. Also, there is a high chance that her daughter will catch it and she may develop a rash within the next 2 weeks.

Answer D2

There is a theoretical risk that Mrs Park is infectious at the moment, so ideally it would be best to see her in a room outside of the antenatal clinic setting.

"Hello Mrs Park, my name is Dr Nobody. I spoke to your community midwife last week and she has explained what happened and why you are so concerned. I believe that it is now 10 days since you visited your friend. How are you feeling at the moment? Has your headache gone now? (*Enquire about prodromal symptoms and a rash etc.*).

Your blood results have come back from the laboratory. Did the midwife explain that we routinely screen your blood for hepatitis B and HIV? I am pleased to be able to tell you that the results of these tests are fine. However, the results for the chickenpox virus suggest that you have never had chickenpox before. They also show that you do not appear to be immune to German measles (rubella).

From this blood test it is too early to say whether or not you could have contracted the virus, and it is a little too soon for any signs of the infection to appear on you. If you become infected you could be quite poorly and there is a very small risk that it could affect the baby, so we should assume that you might become infected and need to give you an injection today to try and prevent things from happening.

I must reassure you that even if you do get chickenpox, it does not increase the risks of congenital abnormalities like spina bifida and heart problems, but there is a small chance (2–3%) of your baby being affected by a syndrome. When I say 'syndrome' I mean a collection of signs. The congenital Varicella syndrome is rare, but can develop if infection occurs for the first time in the first half of the pregnancy. The baby can be affected in a variety of ways. It might have one small, poorly grown arm or leg (limb hypoplasia), neurological abnormalities (microcephaly, hydrocephalus, cortical atrophy, mental retardation), skin scarring (following dermatome distribution) and eye problems (microphthalmia, chorioretinitis, cataracts, Horner's syndrome). There can also be associations with gut, genital and kidney problems and the baby might be small (growth restricted). If you were to become infected, the risk of having a miscarriage is no different from normal.

As for you, if you get the infection you could be very poorly. Apart from the rash, you could develop pneumonia (affects 10–20%, mortality can be as high as 40%) and, very rarely, could suffer with nerve problems (ataxia).

To try and give you some protection we need to immunize you by giving you an injection (zoster immune globulin – ZIG).

The other thing your results show is that you are not immune to rubella, so at the end of your pregnancy we will need to give you an injection to immunize you against this."

Answer D3

Ideally, zoster immune globulin should be administered within the first 3–4 days of contact (1000 mg IM). This can alter or prevent clinical varicella if given within this time, but the evidence that passive immunization prevents fetal infection and damage (congenital varicella syndrome) is limited. There is some evidence of benefit in adults (not specifically pregnant women) if administered up to 10 days after the initial contact.

The risks associated with its use are minimal. The main side effects include mild pain and redness at the injection site. However, it is a blood product, obtained from human volunteers with high titres, and is associated with the commonly encountered risks of blood products.

The Varicella live attenuated vaccine has also been shown to be safe, but it is not licensed for use in the United Kingdom.

Answer D4

The results suggest that she has not been infected by Varicella zoster. The raised IgG is secondary to the ZIG injection. If there was a primary infection, the IgM level would be raised. She can be reassured that on this occasion she has not been infected.

Answer D5

The fact that IgM has been detected suggests a primary Varicella zoster infection, despite ZIG administration.

The woman needs isolating for the period of infectivity. She should be advised not to attend the antenatal clinic or GP surgery. She will also need close observation because the relative immunodeficiency state of pregnancy might increase her chances of developing one of the life-threatening sequelae of Varicella zoster infection. If the woman developed a rash within 2 days of contact with the community midwife she also should be tested for immunity with its consequences.

An ultrasound scan should be arranged for 17 weeks (5 weeks after infection) at the nearest specialist centre to look for signs of fetal damage. Ultrasonic features such as polyhydramnios, hyperechogenic foci in the liver and hydrops fetalis could be found. Amniocentesis and cordocentesis have a limited value in detection of VZ antibodies.

Although there is not enough evidence to confirm that it works, oral acyclovir is relatively safe in pregnancy (there is a theoretical risk of teratogenicity in the first trimester). If it is commenced as soon as possible after the rash develops it might reduce the severity and duration of the illness.

If there were signs that the baby had been infected then pregnancy termination may need to be discussed.

NB. There is a small chance that the IgM result could be a false positive as there is some cross-reactivity with rheumatoid factor.

Answer D6

In an ideal world the answer would be yes. Although rubella infection is much more teratogenic (85% vs. 2–3%), varicella infection is associated with higher maternal morbidity and mortality. The seronegativity rates within the population are similar (6–11% vs. 3–7%) and there are now vaccines available for both the conditions. The difference in the passive immunity for varicella is that it may be protective to the fetus, and does not have the risks associated with administering rubella vaccine during pregnancy.

Whether you could selectively screen all women who did not recall having had chickenpox compared to screening everybody depends on cost-benefit analysis. Factors such as the cost of the vaccine, the cost of the ELISA kit to test for it, compared to the costs incurred in treating an infected mother and her baby would need to be assessed.

Further reading

Gilbert GL (1993) Chickenpox during pregnancy. *Br. Med. J.* **306**: 1079–1080.

Irving WL (1997) Varicella zoster immunoglobulin should be given after exposure to the virus. *Br. Med. J.* **314**: 226–227.

Royal College of Obstetricians and Gynaecologists (1997) Chickenpox in pregnancy. RCOG Guideline 13. Royal College of Obstetricians and Gynaecologists, London.

Seidman DS, Stevenson DK, Arvin AM (1996) Varicella vaccine in pregnancy. *Br. Med. J.* **313**: 701–702.

Slade R (1998) Infections in pregnancy. In: *Key Topics in Obstetrics and Gynaecology*. BIOS Scientific Publishers Ltd, Oxford.

CIRCUIT 2

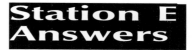

Answer E1

Although unlicensed, the Mirena coil can be used on a named patient basis. In this method the doctor should ensure that

- he/she is adopting a practice that would be endorsed by a responsible body of professional opinion;

- he/she has explained to the woman that this is an unlicensed prescription;

- he/she has explained clearly the perceived risks and benefits, so that informed consent can be obtained and recorded;

- he/she keeps a record of the woman's details and the prescription;

- all practices regarding the product are acceptable to those responsible for the doctor's professional indemnity.

Answer E2

The laser of choice is the Nd:YAG (neodymium:yttrium:-aluminium-garnet) laser. This is the only type of laser that allows destruction of the basal layer of the endometrium, thus achieving a lasting effect.

Endometrial ablation is a highly safe method of treatment with an early postoperative complication rate of 0.77–1.51%. By 6 weeks post-operatively it is 1.25–4.58% and has a mortality rate of only 2 in 10 000. The results of the MISTLETOE study suggest that laser ablation and the roller-ball techniques are the safest. The least safe is a resection with the diathermy loop, but the safety of the procedure increases with the experience of the surgeon.

Ablative methods lead to amenorrhoea or significantly reduced menstrual blood loss in up to 80% of cases in the medium term. They have a lower cost than hysterectomy or long-term medical therapy and allow the avoidance of hysterectomy (and its associated complications) in 80% of women.

Further reading

Irvine GA, Cameron IT (1998) Medical Management of Menorrhagia. RCOG Pace Review 95/ 05. Royal College of Obstetricians and Gynaecologists, London.
Khastgir G, Studd J, Catalan J (1999) Is there a hormonal basis to hysterectomy-related depression? *Br. J. Obstet. Gynaecol.* **106**: 620–622.

Parkin DE (2000) Endometrial ablation techniques. *Obstet. Gynaecol.* **2**: 35–38.

Pinion SB (1994) Conservative alternatives to hysterectomy for dysfunctional uterine bleeding. RCOG Pace Review 94/01. Royal College of Obstetricians and Gynaecologists, London.

RCOG (1999) The management of menorrhagia in secondary care. RCOG Evidence-Based Clinical Guidelines No. 5. Royal College of Obstetrics and Gynaecologists, London.

Richardson RE, Magos AL (1996) Laparoscopic hysterectomy. In: Studd J (ed.), *Progress in Obstetrics and Gynaecology*, Vol. 12, pp. 355–378. Churchill Livingstone, Edinburgh.

Sheth SS (1993) Vaginal hysterectomy. In: Studd J (ed.), *Progress in Obstetrics and Gynaecology,* Vol. 10, pp. 317–340. Churchill Livingstone, Edinburgh.

Slade R *et al.* (1997) Abdominal versus vaginal hysterectomy. *Key Topics in Obstetrics and Gynaecology,* pp. 1–3. BIOS Scientific Publishers Ltd, Oxford.

van den Hurk PJ, O'Brien S (1999) Non-contraceptive use of the levonorgestrel-releasing intrauterine system. *Obstet. Gynaecol.* **1**: 13–19.

CIRCUIT 2

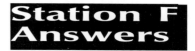

Station F answers

If this scenario is given, you initially need more information about people in order to prioritize them, so conduct a ward round. You need to be able to look at your staff and calculate how best to utilise them.

With regard to Pinker, we need more information. How severe is her pre-eclampsia? Has she been started on the PET protocol? If she has been randomized as part of the MAGPIE trial, I would presume it is severe PET. I would need to know her current observations including her pulse, blood pressure, and urine output (also test for proteinuria). If she were having magnesium sulfate I would need to know about her respiratory rate, tendon reflexes and consciousness level in addition to her urine output. I would like to know what is being used to control her blood pressure and what infusions are currently running – including their rates. The most important thing is to determine how near to delivery is she. Has she come in labouring – if so is she progressing, is the first twin cephalic and why has she not got an epidural sited? Has she been given steroids? If not, it may still be worth giving them now, as they reduce the incidence of intraventricular haemorrhage within an hour. What are her most recent blood results? If not recent, then a full screen will need repeating, looking for HELLP. She may be stable or at high risk. The anaesthetist needs to be involved and the midwife is suitable. The paediatricians need to be informed and preferably introduce themselves.

With regard to Chamberlin, she is a primigravida who is post-term. She has an epidural sited and has been fully dilated for the last 2.5 hours. We need more information, such as has the head been allowed to descend, how long has she been pushing, and is she pushing effectively? What are her contractions like in strength and duration, and does she require syntocinon? What is her partogram like; as she is post-mature, is this a big baby and has she made adequate progress? It would be useful to know the position of the head, and its relationship to the ischial spines. Finally, we need to know about the condition of the fetus. Are the membranes intact, liquor clear and CTG normal?

It is highly probable that if delivery is not imminent she will (if the conditions are appropriate) require an assisted delivery. If this is the case, the anaesthetist may need to top up her epidural and if appropriate the SHO could be asked to assess and deliver her. The midwife is suitable, but her expertise may be required elsewhere and a more junior midwife could be assigned.

In room 2 is Patel. We need more information about her. She has had three consecutive miscarriages and is now 15 weeks pregnant with bulging membranes. At what stage have her other miscarriages occurred – early or mid-trimester? Why is she here on a Sunday for a cervical suture? Was this a planned admission or are there signs of a progressive, further miscarriage? How long have her membranes been bulging – is this long-standing or a recent change? If this is a long-standing problem and she is a planned admission then she can wait. If this is an emergency procedure she is a high priority, but you cannot save a 15-week fetus and she may have to wait.

Jeffcoate has delivered, but her placenta remains *in situ* and she needs suturing. Before I can comment further I need more information. Is she stable or bleeding heavily, either from her uterus or the tear? What were her previous deliveries – has she had a caesarean section to put her at more risk of a placenta accreta? What has been tried to encourage placental separation, has she had syntometrine, is a syntocinon infusion running and what about breast-feeding? If she is not bleeding heavily, then she needs an intravenous line siting and bloods to be sent for a full blood count and group and save. Syntocinon could then be commenced and the anaesthetist informed. If she is bleeding heavily she needs to be consented and taken to theatre for a manual removal and suturing of her tear. This could be done by the SHO. If she delivers the placenta and the tear is small it might be worth asking the community midwife to swap with Jane who could then do the suturing.

We need more information about Shaw. What was the reason for her previous caesarean section, was it a non-recurring (like breech or fetal distress) or was it due to failure to progress? If she had an ARM performed 4 hours ago, was this for failure to progress, as part of an induction or for a non-standard CTG? She should have been re-examined since her ARM so what has her progress been? Why is her progress slow, is this a large baby, an abnormal presentation, inadequate contractions, or a case of cephalo-pelvic disproportion? Is she contracting and dilating adequately or does she require an oxytocin infusion to be commenced? What is the condition of the fetus? Depending on assessment, she may need delivering by a further caesarean section or augmenting. It might be useful to recommend an epidural. The midwife looking after her is suitable.

We need more information about Symmonds. She is a grand multip and if she was 6 cm half an hour ago she might well be about to deliver. I would like to know more about the previous shoulder dystocia. In which pregnancy did this occur and how bad was it (difficult delivery or true dystocia)? Does she have big babies normally? If she normally has large babies and the shoulder dystocia was real then we need to be prepared. She is at risk of a further shoulder dystocia and also a post-partum haemorrhage. Therefore, at a minimum she requires IV access and blood sent to the laboratory for a full blood count and group and save. The senior midwife who is appropriate is looking after her.

Blair is a primigravida who is 30 weeks with presumed ruptured membranes. She needs to be seen by a doctor and assessed and we need further information. Her dates need to be checked and confirmed. She needs a history and examination, especially with regard to her occasional contractions – how strong and frequent? If there is any doubt she should be given steroids immediately. If she appears to be in labour and there are no contraindications then tocolysis should be commenced. The paediatricians will need to be informed and the occupancy of the special care baby unit ascertained, in light of the imminent delivery of 28-week twins. The midwife is appropriate and if she is not contracting and her observations are fine she can be left for the SHO to see later.

Bell in room 7 could also be a problem, but we need further information about her. She is a primigravida post-term, who is being induced for raised blood pressure. She has an epidural sited, has had her membranes ruptured and meconium is draining. She has needed a pH, which was satisfactory. Firstly, how bad is her raised blood pressure, is it mildly elevated or pre-eclampsia? If it is the latter, is she commenced on the labour ward pre-eclampsia protocol and what are her observations like? I would like to know why and when she had her ARM, was it because of an abnormal CTG, as part of her induction or due to lack of progress. If it is due to lack of progress, what has her progress been like recently – are the contractions adequate and does she require syntocinon? We do not know whether the meconium is old or fresh and particulate, and is the CTG abnormal? If the trace was abnormal is it now satisfactory or does she require a further FBS. The pH result alone is not ideal and the full results, including base excess would be desirable. This may need delivering if there is poor progress or further fetal compromise.

Fletcher would appear to be low risk. She has had two previous deliveries and is in spontaneous labour. I would like further information about her in order to make a full assessment. Were her previous deliveries normal or complicated in any way? If she was 3 cm dilated 3 hours ago, when is she due for reassessment? Is she in early labour with irregular contractions or actually established in labour. If she is not in labour and otherwise well, would it be appropriate to transfer her to the antenatal ward until she has established? Sue, the senior midwife is also looking after her, but it might be appropriate to ask one of the other junior midwives like Nicky to take over her care.

Munro is having a termination performed for Down's syndrome at 22 weeks. Theoretically, she should be at low risk, but needs a huge amount of psychological support. I would require more information about her. She is multigravid and presumably having prostaglandins to induce labour. I would like to know whether or not the termination has commenced, and if so how far on she is. If it has not commenced, has she had mifepristone beforehand, if not it might be more appropriate to delay things. She will need a very supportive midwife with good communication skills.

Although room 10 is currently vacant, I would not wish to fill it immediately because there are enough problems and possible problems on the labour ward at present. My priorities would be to ensure the labour ward was stable before potentially creating further problems. Both of the women awaiting further prostaglandins could be assessed on the ward and induced only if there are other indications. The woman with the ruptured membranes can be left, providing that she is asymptomatic with no evidence of chorioamnionitis. Obviously, if there are signs of infection, such as a maternal temperature, tachycardia, vaginal discharge or a raised white cell count she will need to be transferred to the labour ward immediately.

The two problems on the gynaecology ward might be major or minor and again I need further information. The bleeding post-hysterectomy woman might be stable or bleeding heavily, decompensating and requiring an urgent return to theatre. The woman having the miscarriage might be bleeding slightly so she can await a scan (to confirm the diagnosis and exclude an ectopic pregnancy), or be shocked from a massive bleeding and need to go to theatre immediately.

The labour ward is obviously busy, the priorities at present are:

- Pinker – ensure clinically stable and deliver imminently.

- Chamberlin – is delivered or delivering.

- Patel – if not miscarrying can wait.

- Jeffcoate – confirm if placenta still *in situ*, if bleeding heavily then needs theatre.

- Shaw – progress in this labour, perhaps needs a further CS.

- Symmonds – should be delivering shortly, if previous dystocia needs a doctor present.

- Blair – if any evidence of labour needs tocolysis and steroids.

- Bell – ensure clinically stable and fetus OK? Need repeat FBS or delivering.

- Fletcher – if not established and OK transfer to ward.

- Munro – ascertain if termination has started, if not wait.

If the women on the antenatal ward are stable they can wait. If the women on the gynaecology ward are stable they can wait.

The associate specialist should be contacted and asked to come in because an extra pair of hands may be needed. The consultant should be informed of the current situation.

CIRCUIT 2

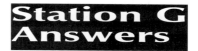

Answer G1

My initial management would depend upon the cause of her problems. First, with regard to her confusion, this could be for several reasons: for instance dehydration, alcohol, raised intracranial pressure and other causes.

The fact that she is dehydrated is noted both clinically and biochemically. She is hyponatraemic and ketotic and will obviously need rehydrating. The reason for her dehydration might well be the vomiting. She is also hypokalaemic. The vomiting could be due to a gastro-intestinal upset, or the fact that she possibly smells of alcohol means that she could have been drinking and has been sick as a result of being drunk. Other causes of her vomiting could be hyperemesis (she has a positive pregnancy test) or secondary to raised intracranial pressure. The rise in intracranial pressure could be as a result of trauma or a space-occupying lesion. This would account for her raised blood pressure, but it is normally associated with a falling pulse rather than a tachycardia, however a tachycardia can occur with dehydration. The proteinuria could indicate a severe urinary infection, which could be a further cause of her vomiting.

The dehydration alone could cause her confusion, but so could alcohol and the raised intracranial pressure.

With a positive pregnancy test and a uterus enlarged to 20 weeks' size she has an intra-uterine pregnancy until proved otherwise. This could be a singleton pregnancy, twin pregnancy or molar pregnancy. The fact that she is bleeding at the moment could suggest a threatened miscarriage or bleeding with a molar pregnancy. If this was a molar pregnancy it could actually be a choriocarcinoma with cerebral metastasis as a cause of her confusion.

Her blood pressure could be raised as a result of her dehydration, raised intracranial pressure or pregnancy-induced hypertension. She could, in fact, be more advanced in her pregnancy with severe PET and a growth-restricted or dead fetus. This might account for the severe proteinuria.

My initial management would be immediate rehydration with IV saline with potassium supplementation. I would examine her myself, including trying to find a fetal heart. I would then arrange an urgent ultrasound scan, ask for a quantitative βhCG. I would send the urine for urgent microscopy and arrange an urgent CT scan of her head. I would ask to speak to the parents as soon as they were contacted.

Answer G2

This shows a mixed sonolucent and echogenic appearance, but no fetus is visible. It is called the 'snow-storm' appearance and is suggestive of hydatidiform mole. The only other things that it could be are a missed abortion or degeneration in a fibroid (but this would not account for the positive pregnancy test).

The diagnosis would be confirmed with an excessively raised serum βhCG level combined with the scan report. The final diagnosis would be confirmed by histological examination of the tissue obtained from the uterus.

The serum βhCG level alone is not diagnostic of molar pregnancy for several reasons. Peak serum βhCG levels in normal pregnancies occur at a time when suspicion of a molar pregnancy usually arises, thus it is only useful after the first trimester (in normal pregnancy serum βhCG reaches its peak levels of 50 000–100 000 IU/l at 8–10 weeks of gestation). Multiple pregnancy can produce similar levels of serum βhCG and only 50% of cases of molar pregnancy produce excessive amounts of βhCG.

Answer G3

The diagnosis is likely to be a molar pregnancy. The excessively high serum βhCG would probably have led to severe hyperemesis causing her dehydration. As well as rehydrating her, I would prescribe an anti-emetic to be given parenterally. I would also be concerned about her blood pressure and consider that this might be pre-eclampsia developing, necessitating anti-hypertensive treatments. The consultant needs to be informed and she needs an urgent uterine evacuation by a senior member of the team. Further bloods need to be taken for cross-matching, to check clotting studies and liver enzymes. I would also repeat her full blood count and electrolytes to note changes since fluid replacement has commenced (her haemoglobin may have been artificially high due to haemoconcentration).

If she has been vomiting persistently she may have become thiamine depleted. If this was the case she could be suffering with Wernicke's encephalopathy accounting for her confusion and nystagmus. She should be given thiamine immediately.

If this is a choriocarcinoma, there is the possibility of cerebral metastasis so an urgent CT or MRI scan needs arranging after thiamine is given.

Answer G4

This is a difficult situation. I would ask the consultant for advice and inform the consultant haematologist and anaesthetist. I may consider talking to my defence organization or the local hospital liaison committee for Jehovah's Witnesses.

Vanessa needs to go to theatre for a uterine evacuation, but due to her level of consciousness she is not sufficiently competent to sign a consent form for the operation. Her condition suggests that she needs this doing quickly because of her high blood pressure, so it would be inappropriate to delay until her consciousness level improves. She could be operated upon without consent because it is a potentially life-saving procedure and is reasonable practice to do so. However, she is at high risk of a uterine perforation and consequent bleeding, which could necessitate a hysterectomy and the need for a blood transfusion.

Talking to her parents about her condition breaches patient confidentiality, but in this case they are still legally responsible for her and can sign the consent form on her behalf. I would explain to her parents that she has a molar pregnancy and needs to go to theatre. I would also explain the risks of the procedure and would ask them to sign a consent form. If they were unhappy to do so we could apply to the High Court for a Specific Issue Order if we felt there was enough time. Otherwise, legally we could operate and give all life-saving treatments (including blood) even if it was against the parents' wishes.

Answer G5

Molar pregnancies are not that uncommon, occurring in the UK in about 1.5 per 1000 live births. There are two distinct types of molar pregnancy – partial and complete (classical). With complete moles there are no embryonal, fetal or placental parts and no amniotic sac. There is gross swelling and proliferation of the syncytiotrophoblasts and cytotrophoblasts leading to central cisternal formation with thin stroma and absent blood vessels, but the villus pattern is maintained. With partial moles the embryo-fetus (usually dead), placenta and amniotic sac are present. There is focal proliferation of the syncytiotrophoblasts with cistern formation and early resorption of the blood vessels.

Genetically, with a complete mole the chromosomes are exclusively derived from the paternal side. The karyotype may be 46XX (commonest), 46XY or 45X. 46XX may be homozygous due to fertilization of an empty or inactivated ovum by a haploid sperm, followed by its duplication (androgenesis). 46XX may also be heterozygous when an empty or inactivated ovum is fertilized by two 23X sperms. 46XY is always heterozygous due to fertilization of an ovum by two different sperms (23X and 23Y).

With a partial mole, the usual karyotype is 69XXY (triploidy). There are two mechanisms for this. Most commonly two sperms fertilize a normal ovum. Alternatively, a normal ovum is fertilized by a diploid 46XY sperm that has failed to undergo normal meiosis. The karyotype may be other than triploid, and not all triploid embryos form partial moles, but in these cases the double chromosomal contribution comes from the maternal side.

With regard to the explanation, I would explain to Vanessa and her parents that it is an abnormal pregnancy, generally caused by one abnormal or two normal sperm fertilizing an egg, and there was no chance that the pregnancy would have continued successfully. I would also explain that it is associated with a 10% chance of residual trophoblastic disease (1 in 200 after partial mole) and a 2–4% risk of choriocarcinoma (1000 times greater than after a normal pregnancy). Thus, we will need to keep a close eye on her for at least the next 2 years (6 months for a partial mole) to ensure it does not recur. To do this we would register her with the most local of the three special units for gestational trophoblastic diseases (Charing Cross Hospital, London, The Jessop Hospital, Sheffield or Ninewells Hospital,

Dundee) for further follow-up. They will monitor her by regular urine (or serum) measurements of βhCG sent by post (42% return to normal in 56 days) every 2 weeks for 6 months. We will also arrange to see her every 6 months for review.

She should avoid another pregnancy for at least 6 months after the serum βhCG levels become normal to reduce the risks of further disease, and because pregnancy makes follow up difficult because of raised serum βhCG. Contraception should be discussed. Barrier methods are recommended because of the theoretical increased risk of metastasis with oestrogen-containing preparations (although there is no evidence to support this). Intrauterine contraceptive devices are avoided as they may cause irregular vaginal bleeding thereby making follow-up difficult.

Hydatidiform mole: *hydatis* (Greek) = a drop of water; *mola* (Latin) = a mass.

Further reading

The Association of Anaesthetists of Great Britain and Ireland (1999) Management of Anaesthesia for Jehovah's Witnesses, London.

Slade R et al. (1998) Gestational trophoblastic disease. *Key Topics in Obstetrics and Gynaecology*. BIOS Scientific Publishers Ltd, Oxford.

Bergin PS, Harvey P (1992) Wernicke's encephalopathy and central pontine myelinolysis associated with hyperemesis gravidarum. *Br. Med. J.* **305**: 517–518.

Davey DA (1995) Normal pregnancy: anatomy, endocrinology and physiology. In: Whitfield CR (ed.), *Dewhurst's Textbook of Obstetrics and Gynaecology for Postgraduates*, 5th edn, pp. 87–108. Blackwell Scientific Publishers Ltd, Oxford.

Fisher PM, Hancock BW (1997) Gestational trophoblastic diseases and their treatment. *Cancer Treat. Rev.* **23**: 1–16.

Howie PW (1995) Trophoblastic disease. In: Whitfield CR (ed.), *Dewhurst's Textbook of Obstetrics and Gynaecology for Postgraduates*, 5th edn, pp. 527–538. Blackwell Scientific Publishers Ltd, Oxford.

Rustin GJS (1992) Trophoblastic diseases. In: Shaw RW, Soutter WP, Stanton SL (ed.), *Gynaecology*, pp. 557–567. Churchill Livingstone, Edinburgh.

CIRCUIT 2

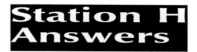

Answer H1

An ultrasound scan should be arranged as soon as possible to make a conclusive diagnosis of fetal death *in utero*. The scan needs to be performed by a person who is skilled as an ultrasonographer, who is able to identify the fetal heart and look for the absence of movements to make the diagnosis. Ideally the person should be able to explain the scan and its findings to the patient. A witness should confirm the death. If I were capable of performing the scan (having undergone the correct training) I would do it myself; otherwise I would accompany the woman to the ultrasound department. The woman should be allowed to see the scan and the lifeless heart.

She may wish to have the scan straight away, wait for her partner or both.

Answer H2

When the ultrasonographer or person performing the scan is satisfied with the reliability of his/her findings these should be shown to the mother (and father). Janice should be told that her baby has died inside her and will need delivering. At this point it may be better to withdraw and leave them alone or to make sure the partner is included, perhaps by suggesting they give each other a hug. The consultant should be informed about the fetal death, and as soon as it is convenient her own GP and community midwife need to be told.

They should be escorted to a quiet, isolated room or area with a supportive atmosphere, preferably away from the antenatal and labour wards. Ideally this room should have an en-suite bathroom, television and basic facilities like a telephone and kettle. There should be adequate space for the partner to sleep. The midwife looking after her or one accomplished as a bereavement counsellor should also be present. The mother (preferably with her partner) should then be counselled about the findings, explaining that the scan is conclusive evidence of the death of their baby. The mode of delivery should also be discussed and a vaginal delivery is often recommended.

It is useful to take time to ask about the events that lead up to the death and ultimately about the whole pregnancy itself. This allows both parents to tell their story and may provide you with the opportunity to explain that they should not blame themselves. (People always want to blame something – it might have been one glass of wine, a piece of soft cheese or an illicit cigarette that now, in the mind of the mother, becomes the reason why she "killed her baby").

It should be emphasized that close co-operation is necessary to ensure a safe labour and delivery. A repeat scan should be arranged if there is any doubt in the mother's mind. All of her questions (and those of her partner) need answering, preferably by a senior obstetrician. It should be made clear that the cause of the fetal death may only be uncovered after the delivery of the baby. Appropriate investigations need to be performed and the couple should be assured that all attempts will be made to achieve a diagnosis, but often no cause is found.

The options available to her are to await labour (expectant management) or to induce it (active management). Both should be discussed and if she so desires, she should be allowed to go home and be given written information (if available) about the management options. Anti-D 500 IU should be given intramuscularly. If she does go home her basic observations (temperature, pulse, blood pressure, and urine) need to be checked first.

(Like most people, I find that breaking this news is the most difficult part of my job. Usually I will hold the mother's, and sometimes father's, hand whilst I am talking to them and will often give both parents a hug. I don't find there is anything wrong with this and the parents often find it comforting to cry on a doctor – AP)

Answer H3

Overall there are no physical disadvantages or advantages in managing the situation actively or expectantly. The main differences relate to their psychological and emotional effects that vary with individuals. The woman and her partner are the best people to choose the method of delivery.

Waiting for the spontaneous onset of labour is of doubtful value in a pregnancy that has lost its goal of a live birth, and obviously the fetus is not deriving any benefit by prolonging the pregnancy. Expectant management is known to be associated with an increased risk of disseminated intravascular coagulation (only after an abruption, otherwise it is rare before 5–6 weeks) and infection. Delayed delivery is also likely to lead to a higher degree of fetal tissue autolysis, so consequently at the time of birth less information can be obtained and questions answered about the possible fetal causes of the death. Psychologically this option may be harder because of the length of time that the woman might be carrying the dead baby for.

On the other hand, expectant management is less invasive with a lower risk of failed induction and other iatrogenic complications.

The methods of induction of labour are prostaglandins alone, normally administered vaginally, the oral antiprogestogen mifepristone, a combination of the two drugs and amniotomy with an intravenous syntocinon infusion.

It is essential to provide adequate analgesia, diamorphine is recommended as a longer lasting and more effective painkiller than pethidine. An epidural can be used if requested (provided there are no contraindications).

Answer H4

A careful examination of a dead fetus can provide some clues as to a possible cause of death. Things that are important include the fetal sex, the size (is it too large or too small), signs of asymmetrical growth restriction, gross fetal oedema and a gross anatomical defect missed by the ultrasound scan. The umbilical cord should be inspected at birth to see if it was wound tightly around the neck or other body parts, whether there was a true knot in it and how many vessels it contains. The placenta might reveal a retroplacental clot, signs of severe placental degeneration or an abnormal insertion of the umbilical cord into it. All of these things can assist in finding the cause of the fetal death; therefore, they should be identified and recorded in the notes.

Parental consent must be obtained prior to requesting any fetal investigations. These include looking for infection by taking swabs from the fetal ear and throat and from the placenta. We need a blood sample (cord and or cardiac blood) for ABO and rhesus typing; karyotyping of the fetal (and placental tissue) is useful. Perhaps the most helpful investigation is a post-mortem examination of the fetus. If the parents do not consent to this then it may be helpful to take a total body X-ray and ask for an external examination of the body and clinical photographs. The post-mortem must be explained both carefully and sympathetically, clarifying its proven values and the fact the baby will be treated with dignity at all times. Even a macerated fetus can reveal anatomical abnormalities that help to define the cause of death (in >33%). The parents should also be informed that tissue will be removed from the body for further histological examination, and this may be stored. They can obviously decline any part of the examination.

Maternal investigations should include tests for metabolic and endocrinological diseases. Thyroid, renal and liver function tests (including bile acids) should be performed (part of the pre-eclampsia screen). There is little evidence to suggest that a fasting blood glucose and Hb A_1C are useful once the baby has died. The only indicator of impaired glucose tolerance might be that the baby is macrosomic. A TORCH screen should be requested and high vaginal and endocervical swabs taken to rule out ascending infection. A Kleihauer and indirect Coombs test may reveal feto–maternal transfusion and subsequent maternal immunization, these should be performed whatever the maternal blood group is. Screening for autoimmune conditions should include assays for anti-cardiolipin, anti-nuclear, anti-Ro, anti-La antibodies, and lupus anticoagulant. Screening for haemotological conditions such as: sickle cell disease/trait, thrombocytopenia (due to autoimmune disease or pre-eclampsia) should be included as part of the investigations. Maternal along with paternal karyotyping is important to detect balanced translocations. Maternal urine toxicological screening should be considered if appropriate.

Answer H5

There are many things that need to be done prior to discharge, and this should not be rushed. The parents should be allowed to go home when and if they feel ready. Although some are physical most are psychological and supportive. It is important to ensure that all investigations have been performed, and a tick list works well for this as an aide memoire.

It is vitally important to allow the parents to see, hold and name the baby. Mementoes (photographs, ink-prints of palms/soles, hair-lock) should be taken for a presentation album. If the parents do not wish to see the baby, their wishes should be respected, but the mementoes should be kept. A blessing by a religious leader should be discussed and arranged if the parents so wish.

Adequate lactation suppression is necessary, either as simple measures or by drug therapy (e.g. Cabergoline or Bromocriptine). The resumption of intercourse and contraception need careful discussion. Information should be provided on self-help groups like SANDS and the Miscarriage Association, and they should be given open access to the team dealing with them. Prior to discharge the general practitioner and the community midwife need to be contacted. It is important to ensure that the appropriate arrangements are made for the funeral ceremony, and method of burial or cremation. The death and cremation certificates require signing.

The couple should be given a follow-up appointment to discuss findings of investigations, provide further help for recovery from the trauma and arrange the management of a future pregnancy. This appointment should be made as soon as the results are available, and if the patients prefer could be in their own home, or a setting away from any pregnant women.

References

Enkin M, Keirse MJNC, Neilson J *et al.* (2000) *A guide to effective care in pregnancy and childbirth.* 3rd edn, pp. 240–243. Oxford University Press, Oxford.

Fox R, Pillai M, Porter H, Gill G. (1997) The management of late fetal death: a guide to comprehensive care. *Br. J. Obstet. Gynaecol.* **104:** 4–10.

Hadlock FP, Deter RL, Harrist RB, Park SK. (1982) Fetal head circumference: relation to menstrual age. *Am. J. Roentgenology* **138:** 647–653.

Hadlock FP, Deter RL, Harrist RB, Park SK. (1982) Fetal abdominal circumference as a predictor of menstrual age. *Am. J. Roentgenology* **139:** 367–370.

Slade R, Laird E, Beynon G, Pickersgill, A. (1998). *Key Topics in Obstetrics and Gynaecology,* 2nd edn. pp. 237–240. Bios Scientific Publishers, Oxford, UK.

Weiner CP. (1996) Fetal death. In: James DK, Steer PJ, Weiner CP, Gonik B. (eds), *High Risk Pregnancy. Management Options,* pp. 1031–1035. WB Saunders Co. Ltd, London.

CIRCUIT 2

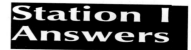

Answer I1

Having introduced myself to Mrs Dean and explained who I am, I would briefly run through the reasons why she is having the laparoscopy. I would enquire about her symptoms to ensure they were still present and to ask about the extent of her pain. I would also ask when her last period was and what she is currently using for contraception. I would then go on to briefly explain the operation thus:

''We are going to have a look inside your tummy with a camera to see if there is any reason why you may be getting your pains. Once you are asleep we make a small cut in your tummy button and place a needle through this. We then fill your tummy with gas. Once this has been done we take the needle out and replace it with a camera, which is about the thickness of my pen. Using the camera we can look at the womb and the tubes and ovaries to see if there is a cause for your problems. If we find anything wrong we would probably be unable to treat it today because we already have lots of other operations to do and would not have the time. Also, it is better to discuss further operations with you once you are awake.

When you wake up your tummy might feel a little sore and you may have some pains in your neck or shoulder. This is because the gas irritates the diaphragm muscle that separates your lungs from your tummy. The nerve supply to this muscle comes from your neck, so that is where the body thinks the pain is.

Very rarely when we do this operation there can be unexpected complications. For example we could damage your bowels or blood vessels. If this happened you could end up with a big cut up and down your tummy and you would be in hospital with us for days, rather than going home tonight.''

I would document in the notes that I have seen her pre-operatively and discussed the operation with its risks to her.

Answer I2

My immediate thoughts are that I have perforated the bowel, either with the Veress needle or the trochar. The fact that I am unable to move the laparoscope from side to side would suggest a trochar injury. I would inform the theatre staff and anaesthetist that this was my concern and try to confirm my thoughts. I would also ask one of the nursing staff to try and contact my consultant to inform him of my worries.

With the laparoscope where it is, I would look again at the left-hand side of the abdomen to try and identify where the faeces is coming from. If I saw faeces I would need to do several things. I would inform the anaesthetist and the nursing staff that we would need to repair the bowel, and I would require assistance for this. The anaesthetist might wish to alter the anaesthetic (e.g. more muscle relaxant, intubate the patient). I would also ask them to cross-match 4 units of blood in case we needed to do a laparotomy. Then I would ask the anaesthetist to give some intravenous antibiotics – a cephalosporin and metronidazole (providing that she was not allergic to any antibiotics). I would also need to consider getting a message to the ward to inform them, because some of the other cases will need cancelling.

If I was uncertain as to whether the trochar was through the bowel I would insert a further trochar suprapubically under direct vision. I would look through this, back up at the umbilical trochar to see if I could see what the trochar had gone through.

Answer 13

The next steps are to contact the consultant who is on call to inform him of the complication. If he is not available, or at his suggestion, I would contact the general surgeon on call for assistance.

Answer 14

If this were the case, I would first inform the theatre staff of the decision to perform a laparotomy, I would then insert a Foley catheter into the bladder, and would immediately re-scrub. I would leave the umbilical port untouched with the laparoscope still through the bowel.

I would then make a midline incision starting beneath the umbilicus and continuing down to about 3 cm above the pubic symphysis. I would incise the sub-cuticular fat to expose the rectus sheath and open this longitudinally. Having identified the linea alba I would divide the recti and carefully open the parietal peritoneum.

If there were extensive adhesions between the abdominal wall and the omentum as previously noted, these might have to be divided to allow access to the abdominal cavity.

I would then search for the entry and exit wounds in the bowel and remove the laparoscope and sleeve. The wounds can be marked by inserting stay sutures at either end. To try and limit further faecal contamination, I would soak a large swab in Betadine and wrap this around the bowel. If the faeces in the abdominal cavity were solid, I would remove it, if liquid I would perform a washout with warm saline containing tetracycline. I would not begin to repair the bowel and would await the arrival of the surgeon.

Answer 15

There are risks associated with any operation. The risks from laparoscopy are well documented, especially with regard to the entry technique. The insertion of a blind Veress needle and trochar into the abdominal cavity is associated with risk of visceral or vessel damage at the rate of about 1 in 1000 laparoscopies.

This was a difficult laparoscopy because the Veress needle was inserted only on the third attempt. The sigmoid colon was adherent to the umbilicus, although there was nothing to have suggested this may have been the case. Even if the technique of open laparoscopy had been used, the bowel may well have been damaged.

The most important aspects of this case are that the risks of damage were discussed pre-operatively and documented, and the damage was recognized immediately and appropriately repaired. Had the damage not been noted then there would be a stronger case for negligence. I would strongly advise that this case be defended.

CIRCUIT 2

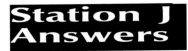

**Station J
Answers**

Answer J1

In this case the indication for the caesarean section in the previous pregnancy is unclear – it could have been fetal distress, dystocia, or cephalo-pelvic disproportion, etc. It would be helpful to get the notes of her previous labour and operation. Assuming it is a non-recurrent indication, and if no other complications occur later in the pregnancy, the chance of a vaginal delivery is good and should be considered to be around 80%. If a vaginal delivery is achieved this time, she will have a good chance of vaginal deliveries in subsequent pregnancies.

Considering the perceived benefits of vaginal delivery, Janet should be counselled appropriately and given the choice of a trial of labour or an elective caesarean section. Overall, attempted vaginal delivery after one section is associated with lower rates of complication for both mother and baby. The morbidity associated with a successful vaginal delivery is 20% of that associated with a repeat section. The risks to the fetus are similar regardless of route of delivery.

However, it is important to make clear to her that in the case of a trial of labour, vaginal delivery is not guaranteed and an emergency caesarean section may become necessary. Failed trials of labour are associated with almost double the morbidity of a planned section, and if she has a further section it is likely that all subsequent babies will be delivered this way (although the evidence to back this up is lacking).

Janet should be warned that the indication for an elective caesarean section might occur in late pregnancy (like a breech), therefore a review of this decision in the late third trimester would be appropriate.

If she wanted to discuss the risks of caesarean in more detail I would explain that there is a four-fold increase in the risk of death (4/10 000) when compared with vaginal delivery. The risks of scar dehiscence are similar (about 2%) and overall maternal morbidity is higher with a section. This is due to the anaesthetic risks, haemorrhage, thromboembolism, infection, operative injury and post-operative pain. I would also reassure her that vaginal delivery is better for the baby because caesarean sections are associated with higher rates of respiratory distress syndrome and fetal anaemia.

I would also explain to her that epidurals are safe in labour, should she require one.

Answer J2

The methods currently available to assess the risk of the cephalo-pelvic disproportion (CPD) are pelvimetry and ultrasonic fetal biometry in late pregnancy.

Pelvimetry (using lateral view pelvic X-rays, CT scan, or MRI scans) is performed in the puerperium and/or late in a subsequent pregnancy. These investigations could be regarded as being of some value only in the case of a cephalic presentation of the fetus in the index pregnancy. Even in this case, their predictive value is significantly reduced due to increased mobility of the pelvic joints in pregnancy and the ability of the fetal head to mould. X-ray pelvimetry in pregnancy has been shown to be associated with a small increase in the risk of childhood cancer, especially leukaemia, which limits its use. A CT scan uses lower doses of radiation, but is more expensive, as is MRI. The latter is not associated with ionizing radiation, so is theoretically safer. However, these two screening methods are not as readily available as X-ray pelvimetry.

Neither X-ray nor clinical pelvimetry have been shown to predict CPD with sufficient accuracy to justify elective sections.

Ultrasonic fetal biometry with subsequent estimation of its weight gives an error of estimation around 10% of the actual fetal weight, which increases at both ends of the range, thus making this also an inaccurate predictor.

Due to these limitations, a carefully monitored trial of labour remains the best method to make diagnosis of the CPD.

Answer J3

There are many causes of a raised AFP, some physiological (twins) and some pathological (neural tube defects, anterior abdominal wall defects, etc.). The best thing to arrange is a detailed anomaly scan, looking in particular at the anterior abdominal wall, especially around the cord insertion, spine, cerebellum (Arnold-Chiari malformation), cranial vault and ventricles. Twins have already been excluded. Some people argue that an amniocentesis should be performed, but there are reports of higher rates of miscarriage when associated with raised AFP.

Answer J4

I would explain that the scan has revealed that the wall of the baby's tummy has not closed over (the gut has actually not returned into the abdomen at 10 weeks of embryonic life) and this is allowing the contents inside the tummy to grow outside. It is a rare condition that occurs in about 1 in 5000 births. I would explain that there is an increased risk of the baby being affected with trisomy 18, and that there is an association with congenital heart defects (10–15%). In view of this I would recommend a further detailed cardiac scan in a few weeks and an amniocentesis.

I would then explain to her that if further investigations are negative, the child should not be born severely handicapped. I would recommend delivery in a tertiary referral unit with a special care unit and access to paediatric surgery. I would arrange a visit and consultation with a paediatric surgeon. They could discuss what is involved with the surgery, the timings after birth, and the risks associated with doing it. I would also arrange a visit to the special care unit in order for the parents to see how it runs, talk to the staff and inform the neonatologists of the future arrival of the child.

Answer J5

Apart from the known anatomical defect, there do not appear to be any other indications for a caesarean section. Babies affected with an omphalocele can be delivered vaginally. However, if this were to be the case I would suggest a planned induction with full paediatric support. The delivery should be in the unit with immediate access to the paediatric surgeons.

Progress of labour, the integrity of the scar and fetal well-being should be monitored throughout. The assessment of the regularity and the strength of the uterine contractions, the rate of dilatation of the cervix and the descent of the presenting part are used for monitoring the progress of labour. During labour she will need to be continually monitored with a CTG.

The assessment of the integrity of the uterine scar is largely associated with the assessment of fetal well-being. The signs of a threatened or partial dehiscence being suprapubic pain (persisting between the contractions), scar tenderness on palpation, and a maternal tachycardia. Partial or complete dehiscence of the uterine scar may present with signs of fetal distress – tachycardia, prolonged decelerations, cessation of uterine activity, disappearance of the fetal head from the pelvis, and readily palpable small parts of the fetus through the abdominal wall. It is important to bear in mind that fetal well-being could also be compromised for reasons independent of scar dehiscence.

There are no restrictions in the use of analgesia – all types are safe. An epidural block is advisable as the risk of caesarean section for this woman is higher than average for the population and it is likely that her unpleasant experience from the previous labour was partly due to her perceived and experienced pain. An epidural may also avoid the use of a general anaesthetic even if an emergency caesarean section becomes necessary. Uterine dehiscence is unlikely to be missed, because the associated pain breaks through all types of analgesia (including epidurals). However, it should be borne in mind that fetal heart abnormalities may occur due to the analgesia and these need to be differentiated from those due to scar dehiscence.

There are no prospective RCTs showing that the use of prostaglandins or syntocinon in women with a scarred uterus increase the risks of rupture or dehiscence. Both agents can be used for induction or augmentation; however, caution should always be exercised. It is logical to use syntocinon to achieve average contraction strength for normal labour with simultaneous continuous CTG monitoring, and monitoring maternal vital signs and the progress of labour.

Further reading

Enkin M, Keirse MJNC, Neilson J *et al.* (2000) *A Guide to Effective Care in Pregnancy and Childbirth*, 3rd edn, pp. 360–371. Oxford University Press, Oxford.

Collis RE, Morgan BM (1995) Regional anaesthesia and obstetrics. *Curr. Obstet. Gynaecol.* **5**: 91–97.

Dickinson JE (1996) Previous cesarean section. In: James DK, Steer PJ, Weiner CP, Gonik B (eds), *High Risk Pregnancy. Management Options*, pp. 207–216. WB Saunders Company Ltd, London.

RCOG (1994) Pelvimetry – clinical indications. The RCOG Guideline No 14. Royal College of Obstetrics and Gynaecology, London.

CIRCUIT 3

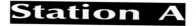

Question A1

This is a referral letter from a GP and a copy of the menstrual chart he gave the patient (next page).

Dr R.J.A. Scotland. MB. ChB. DRCOG

The Schoolhouse Surgery
Muppet Lane
Nowhere-in-particular

The Consultant Gynaecologist
The Cottage Hospital
Nowhere-in-particular.

Dear Dr,

Re: Claire Handcox   Aged 35
Hilltop House, George Street, Nowhere-in-particular

I would be grateful if you would see this difficult lady at your earliest convenience. I have been trying to treat her bloating and heavy periods for some time now, but nothing seems to work. Each time she sees me she is getting more frustrated and angry. She says that not only does she feel like killing her husband, she also feels like killing me! I am sure that she is depressed and possibly has a personality disorder and would appreciate your help as soon as possible. I have given her a menstrual chart to keep her going until she sees you. The only thing of note is a spontaneous venous thrombosis when aged 22. With best wishes,

Yours sincerely

Dr Scotland

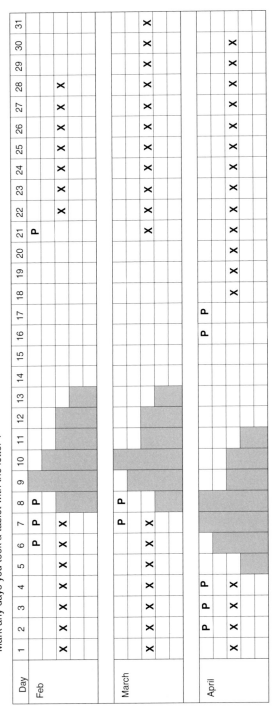

NAME: *Claire Handcox*

MENSTRUAL CALENDER

Key

Mark days of bleeding by shading the boxes, the more boxes, the greater the intensity

Mark any days with pain by using the letter P   Mark any days of other symptoms with the letter X

Mark any days you took a tablet with the letter T

X = Headaches, breast tenderness, bloating

Comment on the chart – what information does it give you?

Your answer here ....

Question A2

From talking to her, her main concern is not her heavy periods but her other symptoms, specifically irrational behaviour, aggression and bloating pre-menstrually. What do you think she is suffering from?

Define the condition and its prevalence. How could your diagnosis be confirmed and the severity of the condition assessed?

Your answer here ....

Question A3

You feel that she is suffering from pre-menstrual syndrome. Describe (in your opinion) the most effective medical treatment modalities for her, and how they might work.

Your answer here ....

Question A4

During your consultation with her you discover that she has a list of over 70 drugs that she has tried to help her condition, none of which has been effective.

What other treatment options are available to her? What else would you like to know before embarking on surgery?

Your answer here ....

CIRCUIT 3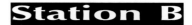

Question B1

What do you understand by the terms medical audit and the audit cycle?

What is the difference between Medical and Clinical audit? Which would you advocate?

What do you mean by audit of structure, process and outcome?

Your answer here ....

Question B2

Design an audit to investigate the outcomes following labour induction in your hospital. Illustrate the type of data you may wish to collect.

Your answer here ....

Question B3

Some of the results of your audit are available and are as follows:

Number of deliveries	2000	
Number of inductions	300	(15%)
Indication for induction:		
Post-term		
> 40 weeks	80	(26.7%)
> 41 weeks	50	(16.7%)
> 42 weeks	20	(6.7%)
Pre-eclampsia	35	(11.7%)
Diabetes	16	(5.3%)
Other maternal conditions	4	(1.3%)
Twins	2	(0.65%)
IUGR	5	(1.7%)
Other fetal condition	2	(0.65%)
Fetal abnormality	4	(1.3%)
FDIU	4	(1.3%)
Maternal request	78	(26%)

Person making decision to induce	
Midwife	1
SHO	15
SpR	99
Staff Grade	151
Consultant	34

Method of delivery		
Vaginal	100	(33%)
Instrumental	50	(17%)
Caesarean section	150	(50%)

Reason for Caesarean section	
Fetal distress	10
Failure to progress	30
Failed induction	110

Methods used	
Membrane sweep	12
Prostaglandins alone	34
Prostaglandins + amniotomy	10
Prostaglandins + amniotomy + oxytocin	185
Amniotomy alone	33
Amniotomy + oxytocin	16
Oxytocin alone	10

What comments would you like to make from this audit?

Your answer here ....

Question B4

What are the benefits of audit?

What is the essential difference between audit and research?

Your answer here ....

CIRCUIT 3

Question C1

Miss Deborah Turner, a 15-year-old schoolgirl, has come to the gynaecology clinic requesting a termination of pregnancy. Her last menstrual period was 8 weeks ago, and her periods are fairly regular. She is studying at the school and does not want to continue the pregnancy.

You are Dr Yaspin Mr Smith's specialist registrar counsel her regarding termination of pregnancy.

[This is a role-playing station, set as a simulated sequence of questions and answers in the gynaecology clinic. Try and answer fully all Miss Turner's questions and concerns. Begin as if you were meeting Deborah for the first time. Her responses are in bold. Ask a friend to role play this Station by reading out the bold type.]

Hello I am Dr Yaspin, Specialist Registrar to Mr Smith. Can I check your name and date of birth please?

Hello I am Debbie. My date of birth is 20th August and I am 15 years old.

Well Debbie, we have had a letter from the family planning clinic telling us that you are pregnant, and that you want this pregnancy terminated.

Yes.

Was this an accident?

Yes, it was the first time we had sex, he promised he would be careful but the condom split. I am studying hard at school you know, and do not want a baby now.

Does your boyfriend know?

No

Do your parents know?

No, I do not want them to know.

Have you talked to anyone at all about this?

Yes, I talked to my friend Sarah's mum. She told me she had an abortion when she was little and it had not done her any harm.

Can I ask why do you not want your parents to know?

I just don't. Dad would go mad, so I don't want to tell them.

It is up to you to decide whether or not you want your parents to be involved. I usually recommend that you tell them, but I'm not going to tell them because whatever you say here and to me will be kept secret. Also, your friend's mum is right; although a termination is a very safe operation most of the time, things can sometimes go wrong. Wouldn't it be a shame if the first thing that your parents knew about you having this operation is that you were very poorly in hospital from a complication of the operation? You never know, they might be more understanding than you think. Also, you will need someone to collect you and escort you home following the general anaesthetic. I must also explain to you that you are only 15, which is under the legal age for giving consent (16 years). It would be better to have your parents support and for them to sign your consent form, although this is not essential.

Debbie, how long have you been seeing your boyfriend?

Not long and he's not really my boyfriend.

OK, so if he's not really your boyfriend who is he?

He's just a friend, alright. Does it really matter who he is?

(Debbie seems to be getting quite upset at this point)

No it doesn't matter who he is. I just want to make sure that you have thought things through and it helps to talk to people. We want you to make the right decision and not to come back and see us again. Why do you want to have the termination?

I'm only a kid, it would ruin my life and my Dad would kill me.

When was your last period, and was it normal?

Yes, it was normal and it was about 8 weeks ago I think.

Are your periods regular?

They come around every month or so. I don't really keep a check on them. Why do you want to know that?

Well, we need to be able to work out exactly how many weeks pregnant you are.

Do you have any problems with your periods, any pain or heavy bleeding?

No, my periods are fine.

Are you quite well otherwise? Do you have any illnesses and have you ever had an operation for anything before?

No, I'm fine otherwise.

Do you take any medicines for any reason?

Only my asthma inhaler.

Do you smoke, drink alcohol or use any illegal drugs?

No

Are you allergic to anything?

No

What contraception are you planning to use after the operation?

Condoms – in the sex lesson at school they told us that condoms prevented AIDS.

Yes, they do but they are more likely not to work when compared to some other contraceptive methods. If you are not in a longstanding relationship it is a good idea to use condoms each time you have sex, but it might also be worth you thinking of other methods of contraception to use at the same time, like the pill.

Before I agree to the termination I will need to examine you. Have you ever had an internal exam before?

No. Why do you have to examine me?

I need to feel exactly how big your womb is before we operate on you, to make sure that it fits with how far on you think you are.

Question C2

You examine her and confirm that she is 8–10 weeks pregnant, consistent with her dates.

Discuss the operation of a termination with her.

Your answer here ....

Question C3

What if you had examined Debbie and found that her uterus was at her umbilicus and a bimanual examination confirms she is about 22 weeks pregnant.

What would you do now?

Your answer here ....

Question C4

What if you had examined Debbie and found that her uterus feels a normal size. What are you going to tell her and what will you do now?

Your answer here ....

Question C5

Returning to the original findings of an 8 week uterus. On what grounds would you agree to perform the termination?

Your answer here ....

Question C6

Debbie leaves you and goes to see Sheila, the counsellor next door. After she has spent half an hour with her, Sheila comes through to you. She informs you that Debbie has broken down in tears and has told Sheila that her 'boyfriend' was actually her father.

What are you going to do?

Your answer here ....

CIRCUIT 3

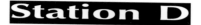

Question D1

The following information leaflet has been written for women prior to visiting a colposcopy clinic. It is sent to them before they attend the clinic. This is a new initiative for the colposcopy clinic.

Read it and comment about it.

Your answer here ....

WELCOME TO THE COLPOSCOPY CLINIC

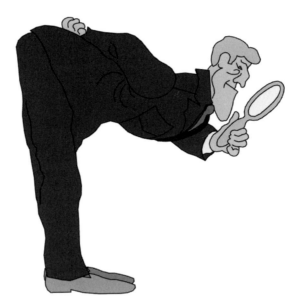

GYNAECOLOGICAL INFORMATION BOOKLET

Written by Dr N.O. Idea
Consultant Obstetrician and Gynaecologist

The smear test

Your doctor has referred you to the colposcopy clinic following the results of your cytological screening test. When you have cytological screening the cytologists examine the exfoliated squamous epithelial cells from your ectocervix and the glandular cells from your endocervix. They look at these for abnormalities, such as increased mitotic activity and abnormal nuclear to cytoplasm ratios. They can then try to grade these cells depending on how abnormal they look. The result from your test may have shown only slight abnormalities (mild dyskaryosis) through to micro-invasive cancer. The test may also have revealed that you are infected with the wart virus (human papilloma virus), which may be contributing to the abnormalities.

Your first visit to the colposcopy clinic

The smear test is not that accurate in determining exactly what is going on in the cells in the cervix, so that is why you need a colposcopy. Colposcopy involves looking at the cervix (neck of the womb) with a special large microscope. This is often connected to a television set so you and everyone else in the room can see what is happening. This is a teaching hospital, so there are often trainee doctors, nurses and medical students observing the colposcopy and attending the clinics. If you really do not want them there you must immediately inform the doctor when you meet him and they will be forced to leave.

When you come to the clinic you will be met by a doctor, who may be strange to you. He will tell you to get undressed and change into a gown. Then he will ask you a lot of questions about things as diverse as your parity, smoking habits and sexually transmitted diseases. You will then be escorted by a nurse to the colposcopy couch. This is a specially designed bed to make you feel as comfortable as possible whilst having your innermost parts examined. You will be asked to put your legs up in stirrups and have them strapped in. The doctor will then move the colposcope in between your legs. It is very important to be relaxed during the entire procedure otherwise it will hurt more.

The doctor will then take another smear to compare it with the first one and his findings for the purpose of audit. He will then look very carefully at the neck of the womb for any mild abnormalities and signs of cancer or pre-cancer. He will then paint the neck of the womb with different solutions. The first one is an acid (acetic acid) that shows up the pre-cancerous cells as white areas – you should be able to see these changes on the television screen. He might then apply iodine (a brown dye) to confirm these changes. Abnormal cells do not take up this dye and even if the doctor has missed the more subtle changes with the acid he should be able to detect any abnormalities this way.

If he sees any abnormalities he will want to take a biopsy from those areas. A biopsy means removing a piece of tissue from the body. This can be sent to the histopathologists to be compared with the cytological findings. The biopsy or biopsies are obtained using sharp pincers that cut into the cervix to remove the tissue. We do not usually use any anaesthetic for this and it does not normally hurt very much.

The site of the biopsy may bleed so the doctor will use silver nitrate sticks to try and seal the blood vessels before you can go home. You should bring a sanitary pad with you just in case you bleed heavily.

Your second visit to the clinic

It is very likely that you will need to come back to the clinic for your results. The results normally take 2 weeks to come back to us from the cytologists and histopathologists. Depending on what grade of CIN or cancer they may show will determine how we subsequently manage you.

If your results show cancer, do not worry because it is likely that we can cure you with a radical hysterectomy, where we remove the womb and the lymph nodes to which any cancer may spread. If the cancer has spread you would then require radiotherapy (not the treatment that makes you lose your hair) to try to cure you.

If the biopsy shows CIN 2 or 3 you will require further treatment with a LLETZ. With this technique we pass an electric current through a wire which we move across your cervix while you are awake. This removes a loop of tissue and is normally the only treatment you may require. Sometimes we have to do a cone biopsy where we use a special knife to cut the abnormal area away. You would be asleep for this.

If we perform the large loop excision of your transformation zone (LLETZ), we use the colposcope to define the abnormal areas, and before we do the treatment we inject lots of local anaesthetic through many needle-pricks into the neck of the womb. Usually, although not always, this freezes the neck of the womb and you will not feel any pain. We connect you to the electricity generating machine by placing a large pad on your leg. This is essential to allow the equipment to work and to prevent you from getting any burns. You will hear noises as we use the equipment, and although we use a vacuum pump you may smell the burning caused by the electric current. To try to stop you from major bleeding we then heat-seal the blood vessels.

Very rarely there can be complications such as major haemorrhage – sometimes requiring admission to the hospital, taking you back to theatre and blood transfusions. It is more common to get an infection afterwards which causes bleeding. To try and reduce the chances of you having any bleeding you should not use tampons or have sex after you have had the treatment done. There is an association with cone biopsies and infertility, late miscarriage and painful periods, but this does not seem to be the case with the LLETZ.

If the biopsy shows CIN 1 we do not necessarily have to undertake a LLETZ, but you will need further surveillance because CIN 1 may progress to more invasive disease and can be associated with more invasive disease in the surrounding area.

In most cases after a colposcopy and minor treatment, you should be able to go back to work the following day. We do not advise that you return to full activities for 6 weeks afterwards.

We look forward to seeing you soon.

If you require any further information please do not hesitate to write to us at the hospital.

CIRCUIT 3

Question E1

As the junior doctor's representative, you are asked to join the obstetric risk management team. One of the main jobs that the team is tasked with is to react to clinical incidents and try to minimize litigation. You are asked to look through documents relating to a case that occurred a couple of years ago.

What comments would you like to make?

Your answer here ....

DOCUMENT 1 – SOLICITOR'S LETTER

LOWEST OF THE LOW

Mr Really Stupid
Chief Executive
No Hope Hospital
Wiltshire

Solicitors and Barristers
The Chambers Pot
Loo Street
Wiltshire

April 1st

Dear Mr Stupid

Re: Miss Evelyn Primrose
     Flat 102, The Stacks, Warminster

I am writing on behalf of my client Miss Evelyn Primrose who is instituting legal proceedings against your hospital. She alleges negligence in your duty to care for her during her pregnancy and the delivery of her second child Kylie. She is now 2 years old and is showing signs of developmental delay. She also has limited use of her left hand following a negligent delivery.

She alleges that:

1. You failed to advise her of the risks of poor control of her diabetes and did not adequately monitor or treat the condition.

2. You should have realized that Kylie was a large baby and delivered her by an elective Caesarean section, instead of putting her through a prolonged labour.

3. Had you delivered Kylie by Caesarean section she would not have sustained the injuries to her humerus and clavicles.

4. Had a Caesarean been performed she would not have shown developmental delay.

5. The delivery has resulted in the development of urinary incontinence, which is severely embarrassing and debilitating. A Caesarean section would have prevented this from occurring.

We await your response.

Yours sincerely,

DOCUMENT 2 – COPY OF THE REFERRAL LETTER

Dr N.O. Idea
The Peak Practice
High Contraction
Umbilical Road
Warminster

Dr Diane Bettic
Consultant Obstetrician
No Hope Hospital
Mortis Lane
Wiltshire

Dear Dr Bettic

Re: Miss Evelyn Primrose
Flat 102, The Stacks, Warminster

This 22-year-old girl finds herself pregnant again. It is only 15 months since the birth of her son Jason. She came to see me last week requesting a depo injection. She had been using Depo-Provera since Jason was born, but had not reattended for her repeat injection 6 months ago. I examined her and was surprised to find her uterus at the level of the umbilicus. I sent her for a scan that has shown an 18-week sized pregnancy. She asked me for a termination, but I explained that I would not be willing to support this, and I suggested referring her to the private clinic in the city. She thought about it but has come back and decided to have the baby.

You might remember her; she is only short (about 5 feet 3 inches), but weighs 116 kg. She is a very poorly controlled diabetic, who, after a long and abusive last labour, produced Jason weighing 4.1 kg. As you were so nice to her last time, she has asked to see you again. I checked her HbA$_1$C last week and this was 7% (normal laboratory range – upper limit 4.9%). She wishes to be sterilized after the delivery.

Yours sincerely,

Dr N.O. Idea

DOCUMENT 3 – COPIES OF GROWTH SCANS

**GRAPH OF HEAD CIRCUMFERENCE VS.
GESTATIONAL AGE
(after Hadlock et al, 1982c)**

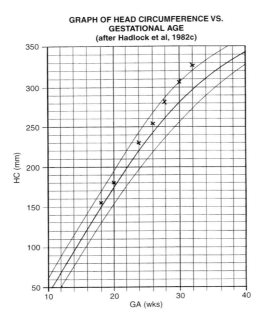

**GRAPH OF ABDOMINAL CIRCUMFERENCE VS.
GESTATIONAL AGE
(after Deter et al, 1982)**

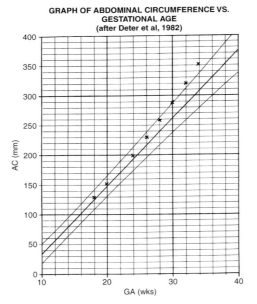

DOCUMENT 4 – COPY OF THE PARTOGRAM

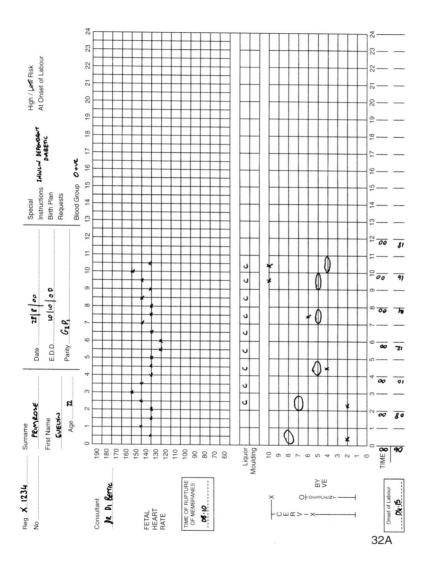

32A

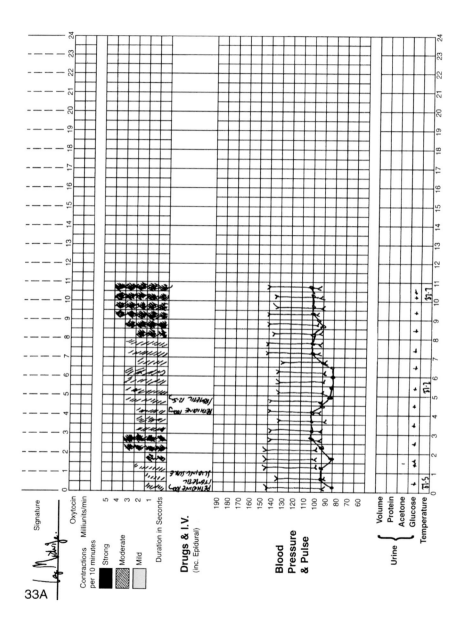

33A

DOCUMENT 5 – DISCHARGE SUMMARY

NO HOPE HOSPITAL

OBSTETRIC AND NEONATOLOGY DIRECTORATE

DISCHARGE SUMMARY

MOTHER:

	Evelyn Primrose	X1234
	Admitted	28/08/00
	Discharged	30/08/00

Antenatal problems	Poorly controlled insulin-dependent diabetic – despite repeated advice and joint management with the diabetologist each week. Previous admission for pre-term labour
Delivery	Spontaneous onset at 34 weeks Neville Barnes forceps
Complications	Shoulder dystocia Extended episiotomy – third degree tear
Medications	Codeine, lactulose, ferrous sulfate, Augmentin
Follow up	Hospital post-natal clinic 6 weeks

BABY: Kylie Primrose   Sex: Female   Born 28/08/00
Weight 4.123 kg

Kylie was admitted to the SCBU following a traumatic vaginal delivery.
Problems: Prematurity (34 weeks)
1. Mild RDS – needed ventilation for 7 days
2. Small intraventricular haemorrhage
3. Physiological jaundice
Macrosomia
1. Left brachial plexus injury – resolved
2. Left humerus and both clavicles fractured
3. Hypoglycaemia
4. Suspected diabetic cardiomyopathy and SVT
Hypotonia – persisting

Discharge medications: Folic acid 1 mg weekly
Flecainide 4 mg tds
Abidec 0.6 ml od
Follow-up: Paediatric cardiology clinic 2 weeks

DOCUMENT 6 – ENTRY IN THE NOTES REGARDING DELIVERY

28.8.00

18.15 Called to see by midwife
34/40 diabetic, pushing for 1 hour with little progress
CTG – early decelerations, becoming more prolonged
VE: Fully dilated, moulding, caput, ?OA
      Forceps applied
      Head delivered with 3 pulls
      RMLE
      Shoulders stuck – reg. called.

Felix Stuck

18.20 Crash called by midwife
Shoulder dystocia following forceps
Legs already in lithotomy
Episiotomy extended
Difficult delivery of shoulders
? fracture
Episiotomy repaired in layers with adequate local
Third degree tear oversewn.
Stop sliding scale
Transfer to ward

Justin Time (Reg.)

Question E2

What do you understand by the term 'clinical risk management' and do you feel that it leads to practising defensive medicine?

Your answer here ....

Question E3

Why it is a part of clinical governance?

Your answer here ....

Question E4

What are the fundamental principles of CRM? Do you think CRM can eliminate litigation? Overall, how can malpractice be reduced?

Your answer here ....

Question E5

What human factors are responsible for clinical adverse events?

Your answer here ....

CIRCUIT 3

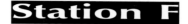

Question F1

You are called to the delivery ward by your SHO, who has just performed a Neville Barnes forceps delivery on Evelyn Primrose and he cannot deliver the baby's shoulders. The indication for the forceps was poor maternal effort following pushing for an hour at full dilatation, and the development of early decelerations on the CTG. After being placed in the lithotomy position and cleaned and draped, the fetal head was delivered after three pulls, and a right mediolateral episiotomy had been performed. One minute later the midwives call you (as the second on call for the labour ward) because the fetal shoulders have not yet delivered.

What are you going to do?

Your answer here ....

Question F2

Baby Primrose is safely delivered. Unfortunately, it was a difficult dystocia and you finally removed her by grasping the posterior arm. During the procedure you broke the left humerus and clavicle. The baby appeared to hold its left hand backwards, in the 'waiters tip' position. Evelyn and her partner are quite angry about the delivery and wish to be 'de-briefed'. Your consultant said he would go and see them personally, but is still tied up in a meeting. The midwives ask you to go instead.

What would you say to them?

Your answer here ....

Question F3

How might you have improved the outcome for this baby?

Your answer here ....

CIRCUIT 3

Question G1

Vicky Beck is a 29-year-old woman, who has been married for 3 years to David and has been trying for a pregnancy for the last 2 years without success. Her GP has not investigated them, but has referred them directly to the gynaecology clinic. Mrs Beck has come today to see Dr Jaffas (the consultant in your unit with an interest in infertility) with her husband. The couple are both very anxious about their lack of conception. You are Dr Alistair Davies, Dr Jaffas' specialist registrar and you have been working with him for the last 5 months.

Please talk to the Becks. Initially take a short infertility relevant history and then counsel them about initial investigations.

[This is a role-playing station, set as a simulated sequence of questions and answers in the gynaecology clinic. Try and answer fully all Mrs Beck's questions and concerns. Begin as if you were meeting her for the first time. Her responses are in bold. Ask a friend to role play this Section by reading out the bold type.]

Hello, Mr and Mrs Beck, my name is Alistair Davies. I am Dr Jaffas' registrar. I need to ask you a few questions and then we can have a chat about things.

How old are you Mrs Beck?

Hello, we are pleased to meet you, we have been ever so long waiting for this appointment and we are so glad that we are here. I am Victoria Beck. I am 29 years old.

How old are you Mr Beck?

Hello Doctor, I am 55 years old.

How long have you been trying to get pregnant?

We have been trying for a baby for the last 2 years without any success. I am really anxious to know whether I am able to conceive naturally at all.

Have you ever been pregnant Mrs Beck?

No, never.

Have you any children Mr Beck?

Yes, I have been married before and I had two children with my wife. They are both in their early twenties now and I hardly ever see them.

Do any of the children live with you?

No.

How long have you been married or living together?

We have been living together for 5 years and married for 3 years.

Are your periods regular?

Yes, every month.

When was your last one?

Two weeks ago

Are they heavy or painful?

No

Do you have any other pains ever?

No, occasionally I feel a little uncomfortable in the middle of the month and I presume that is when I am ovulating.

Do you have any pains or problems with intercourse?

No, well not all the time, but occasionally it hurts.

Does it hurt on the inside or the outside?

Deep on the inside, sometimes we have to stop.

Is the pain associated with any particular time of the month or sexual position?

No, not that I have noticed.

Do you have intercourse regularly?

Most of the time, however David travels a lot and is often away on business.

Do you have any vaginal discharge, and have you ever had any sexually transmitted diseases?

No, certainly not.

What have you used in the past for contraception?

I was on the pill for many years, but stopped taking it 3 years ago, just after we got married. We then used condoms for 6 months before we decided the time was right for a baby.

Are you up to date with your smears, and have they ever been abnormal?

My last smear was last month and it was fine. I did have some abnormal cells treated when I was at college. I had a cone biopsy to sort them out. All my smears since have been OK.

Do you know how abnormal the cells were?

No, they just said they were pre-cancerous.

Have you ever suffered from any serious illnesses or had any operations?

No.

Are there any diseases that run in the family, or have there been any abnormal babies born?

No.

Do you take any medications or drugs for any reason?

No.

Do you smoke and drink alcohol?

Yes, about 20 a day and we have a glass of wine most nights.

Do you both work?

Yes, I work in a food factory packing spices and David is a long distance lorry driver.

David, are you generally in good health?

Yes

Have you ever had any operations or problems with your testicles?

No

Do you smoke and drink alcohol?

Yes, about 20 a day and we have a glass of wine most nights when I am home. I buy it cheap from France.

Do you take any medications or drugs for any reason?

No.

Have you had any investigation or treatment for this problem?

No. We went to see our doctor who referred me to the hospital. I really don't understand where we are going wrong.

Counselling

Let me try to explain things to you a little now. About one in 10 couples have problems getting pregnant. For a pregnancy to occur, a normally functioning sperm must reach the fallopian tube to meet a normally functioning egg. The sperm-head enters the egg and creates the earliest form of a baby called an embryo. The embryo travels into the womb within about 4 days and then begins to bury into the lining of the womb. The baby then grows over the next 9 months.

There are several things needed for this to occur. First, the man needs to be able to produce good quality sperm and they need to be able to get from the vagina, through the neck of the womb into the centre of the womb. They then need to be able to get down an open fallopian tube in order to meet the egg and fertilize it. Obviously, the other thing that needs to happen is that the woman produces an egg each month. Hormones are important for this to occur, and they need to be produced in a certain order.

Any problem preventing these things from happening may prevent a pregnancy from occurring. Generally speaking, female factors are present in about half of cases, male factors are responsible for about a quarter of cases and the rest are due to a combination of factors. Overall, the causes of infertility are unexplained (27%), male factors (24%), anovulation (20%), tubal factors (14%), endometriosis (6%), sexual dysfunction (6%) and cervical (3%).

What could be the problem in our case?

I need to examine both of you first and then arrange for some tests to check David's sperm quality, whether you are ovulating or not and your rubella status. There could be several reasons why you are not getting pregnant. The first may be just one of practicalities – because David is away so much you may be missing the time that the egg is released each month. Men who are long-distance lorry drivers may have a lower sperm count because as they spend so long sitting down, the testicles get pushed nearer to the body and they warm up. The result of this is lower sperm production. Alcohol and smoking can also affect sperm counts.

The other things we need to think about are the fact that you have previously had a cone biopsy. The cervix produces mucus that is beneficial in protecting sperm, operations on the neck of the womb like cone biopsies can alter this and this could be contributing to your lack of success in getting pregnant.

Another thing you mentioned was pain with intercourse. Occasionally this can be due to endometriosis, a very common condition that can cause or be associated with infertility. It might be best if we look inside your tummy with a camera, an operation called a laparoscopy. We can look at your fallopian tubes to see if they are open, and look for any signs of endometriosis because of your pains.

Are there any other ways of checking my tubes?

Yes, we could arrange for an X-ray called a hysterosalpingogram, or HSG. The radiologist inserts a small tube into your womb and injects dye through it. They can then take some X-ray pictures to watch where the dye goes. This also allows us to look at the inside of the womb to make sure there are no polyps or fibroids there. Another way is to use an ultrasound scan – called a HyCoSy. Here we also put a small tube into the womb and inject dye through it, but we use a scan rather than X-rays to see whether or not the tubes are open. However, both of these tests do not allow us to look and see whether or not you have endometriosis. The only way of telling that is by a laparoscopy.

How do you check for ovulation?

The only time we actually know that you have ovulated is when someone gets pregnant. All of the other tests we do look for changes suggestive of ovulation. The commonest test we do is a blood test 21 days after the start of your menstrual cycle. We only use day 21 if your periods are 4 weeks apart; otherwise we do the test 7 days before the expected date of the period. In this test the levels of the hormone progesterone are checked. Progesterone is produced only in the ovary; it starts to rise a little just before the egg is released and may play a role in starting ovulation. However, once the egg has been released the levels of progesterone climb steeply. Its job is to alter the lining of the womb to get it ready to accept an embryo if one comes. A normal day 21 progesterone level does not mean that ovulation has definitely occurred with the release of the egg, but it suggests this is the case.

Another way to check for ovulation is to look for another hormone called LH. This is produced by the pituitary gland, a small gland at the base of the brain behind the eyes. It causes changes to occur in the cells around the egg and actually causes ovulation. It is rapidly excreted in the urine, so simple urinary kits can detect it. They are expensive and do not precisely time ovulation, although it usually occurs within 1 or 2 days of the LH being detected.

For ovulation to actually occur, the follicle that contains the egg and some fluid has to burst. In about 10% of menstrual cycles in infertile couples this does not seem to happen, but the unruptured follicle produces the progesterone hormone and the period will occur at the right time. This is called a luteinized unruptured follicle (LUF) and can only be detected by scanning the ovaries throughout the month.

What would you do if I were not ovulating?

We would first need to try and find any reason why this was not the case. If we could not find any particular reason I would give you some tablets called clomiphene. You have to take these for 5 days, starting on the day after your period has started. The tablets increase the chances of producing more than one egg at a time so there is a higher risk of twin pregnancies. Very rarely the ovary can over-respond and you can become quite poorly from ovarian hyperstimulation syndrome.

If you did not appear to ovulate, initially we would increase the dose of clomiphene. If you did not ovulate even after 6 months we would refer you to the infertility clinic for further management. The reason for this is that we cannot recommend using clomiphene for a long time because prolonged use of clomiphene has been seen to be associated with increased risk of ovarian cancer. Hence, the present recommendation is not to use it for more than 6 months.

Question G2

These are the results of the investigations performed.

Semen analysis on David Becks aged 55:

PH	7.5
Volume	5 ml
Sperm concentration	20×10^6/ml
Motility	20% with forward progression
Morphology	30% with normal morphology

Progesterone – Day 21:   34 nmol/l

Laparoscopy and Dye:
Severely stenosed cervix, unable to cannulate.
Laparoscopy revealed minimal endometriosis in both ovarian fossae, the pouch of Douglas and a nodule on the left uterosacral ligament. There was no evidence of adhesions or endometriosis of the ovaries.

HSG: Unable to cannulate cervix.

What do you think of the results and what treatment would you recommend, if anything?

Your answer here ....

Question G3

Three months later, a repeat semen analysis and swim-up is performed and is acceptable for IVF. Vicky has been seen again when menstruating and it has been possible to cannulate her cervix with a fine catheter. Having discussed all the treatment options with you they decide they wish to proceed immediately with IVF and a fresh embryo transfer.

Briefly outline the points that you would discuss with them in an IVF counselling session.

Your answer here ....

CIRCUIT 3

Question H1

A 57-year-old lady comes to the gynaecology clinic complaining of leaking urine while coughing or sneezing for the last year. She also suffers from increased frequency of micturition during the day. At night she usually goes to the toilet once or twice to pass urine. She has to go to the toilet immediately once she feels the urge to void, otherwise she would lose urine. The last two problems started 6 months ago. She had her menopause 8 years ago at the age of 49 and has never used HRT. She has two children; both were average sizes, delivered vaginally after long labours. She is otherwise well, but like her mother suffers with glaucoma.

How would you manage her?

Your answer here ....

Question H2

Why would you arrange urodynamic studies to make a diagnosis, and which single commonly used urodynamic test would be most helpful?

Your answer here ....

Question H3

What is the value of a frequency-volume chart in assessing the type of incontinence? What is the best investigation for assessing detrusor instability (DI), and what would you do if it were reported as normal?

Your answer here ....

Question H4

If urodynamics revealed mixed incontinence what would you do and why?

Your answer here ....

Question H5

What treatments do you know for DI, how effective are they and what would you advise for her?

Your answer here ....

Question H6

What are the treatment options for GSI, how are they performed and how effective are they?

Your answer here ....

CIRCUIT 3

Question 11

Mrs Jones, a 40-year-old woman, has just returned from the ultrasound department following her routine booking scan. It has shown a twin pregnancy.

The comments from the ultrasonographer are that:

- This is a twin pregnancy
- The uterus contains two sacs divided by membranes containing one fetus in each
- Both fetal heartbeats are seen
- The measurements are consistent with her dates (13 weeks)
- One placenta is noted posteriorly
- 4 cm fibroid anteriorly

What type of twin pregnancy is it likely to be? How can you determine that from the scan and why is it important?

Your answer here ....

Question 12

This is a total shock to her, but probably explains the severe heartburn that she is already experiencing, which is not relieved by antacids. She already has two children and this was a spontaneous conception. Her last two pregnancies were uneventful, culminating in normal vaginal deliveries at 39 weeks. She requests midwifery led care and a home birth with this child.

What advice would you give her?

Your answer here ....

Question 13

Mrs Jones declines all screening tests, but reluctantly agrees to your suggestion of shared care. She does not wish for any medical treatment for her heartburn, preferring herbal remedies instead.

You meet her next when 22 weeks pregnant following her routine scan. This shows that the anterior fibroid has grown to 8 cm. The placenta remains posterior and high. The abdominal circumferences are 16 cm for twin 1 and 13 cm for twin 2. The amniotic fluid volume around twin 1 is normal, but there appears to be very little liquor around twin 2.

What would you suspect, why would this concern you and how would you subsequently diagnose and manage it?

Your answer here ....

Question 14

What do you understand by fetal acardia in relation to twin pregnancies?

Your answer here ....

Question 15

Suppose a 30-year-old primigravida has come to see you in the antenatal clinic. She has an ultrasound scan which shows a viable intrauterine twin pregnancy of 7 weeks gestation. What will you tell her?

Your answer here ....

Question 16

How would you manage a case of a diamniotic-monochorionic twin pregnancy at 30 weeks gestation where one fetus is found to be dead?

Your answer here ....

CIRCUIT 3

Question J1

Electrosurgery is a vital part of the equipment used by surgeons. Explain the principles behind the use of diathermy, including the differences between monopolar and bipolar, cutting and coagulation and what factors are essential for its safe use.

Your answer here ....

Question J2

What do you understand by the term suture?

How are different sutures classified, and what are their differences?

Look at the different sutures below, describe them.

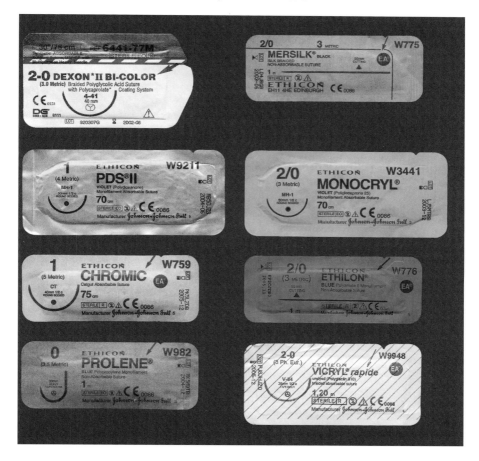

Your answer here ....

Question J3

What are these paired instruments and what would you use them for?

1.

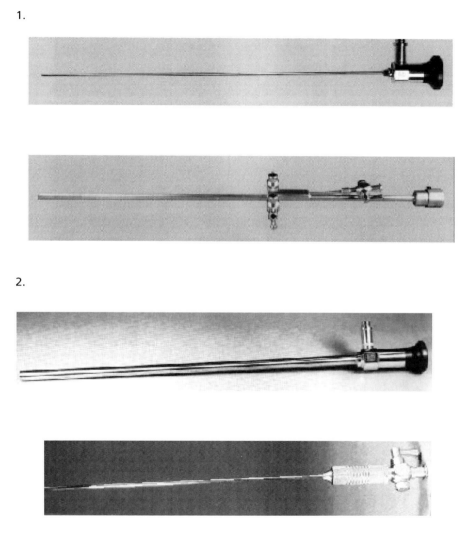

2.

Reproduced with permission of Rimbros Ltd (RB Endoscopy)

Your answer here ....

Your answer here (cont.) ....

CIRCUIT 3

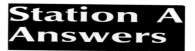

Answer A1

The chart shows that she has a regular menstrual cycle. She bleeds for between 6 and 8 days, her periods appear regular and they occur every 28–29 days. She only appears to have 1–2 days of heavy loss (4/5 shaded boxes) each month. The rest of her menstrual loss seems moderate or light.

She always seems to get pain for 2–3 days before her periods start, and this settles with the beginning of menstruation.

In February and April she also had mid-cycle pain, which may have been 'Mittelschmerz'.

She starts to get other symptoms from day 14–15 and these last until her menses start. She has commented that these are headaches, mood swings and breast tenderness. We do not know the severity of each of the symptoms or whether they all occur together or separately.

Answer A2

I think she is suffering from pre-menstrual syndrome (PMS). PMS may be defined as a cyclical recurrence of non-specific psychological, behavioural and somatic symptoms in the luteal phase of the menstrual cycle, which are relieved by the onset of, or during, menstruation. The symptoms may be severe enough to disrupt the patient's life significantly. The syndrome occurs irrespective of socioeconomic status, race or cultural background.

Although symptoms of premenstrual tension occur in over 90% of women during their reproductive lives, they are severe enough to consult the doctor in 20–40% and are classified as severe and incapacitating in only 2–6%.

PMS should be considered primary if symptoms resolve completely by the end of the menstruation and there is a symptom-free week between the end of the period and the time of ovulation. In contrast, secondary PMS is characterized by only partial resolution of the symptoms by the end of the menstruation. The baseline is the level of prevailing psychogenic disorder.

There are a large number of symptoms described in association with PMS (greater than 150), but these are not specific to, or for PMS. It is the cyclical occurrence of the symptoms that are specific for the disease. Therefore, the diagnosis of PMS should be based on prospectively administered symptom-rating charts for at least two cycles. These may reveal the occurrence of the symptoms, the degree of underlying psychopathology and the extent to which the condition disrupts the patient's life.

The commonest symptoms are emotional and behavioural, including depression, irritability, lability, anxiety, poor concentration, change in libido, aggression or violence, food cravings, fatigue and loss of self-control. Physical symptoms include breast tenderness and swelling, bloating, acne, swollen fingers and ankles, backache, weight gain, and headaches. There may also be exacerbations of chronic illnesses such as asthma, migraine and epilepsy.

The involvement of psychiatrists and the use of the GnRH analogue test should be considered where the clinical diagnosis is difficult.

The diagnosis according to the *Diagnostic and Statistical Manual of Mental Disorder*, third edition, revised (DSM-III-R):

A: In most menstrual cycles in the past year the symptoms listed under (B) occurred during the last week of the luteal phase and disappeared again a few days after onset of the follicular phase. In menstruating women this phase corresponds to the week before and a few days after the start of menstruation.

B: At least four of the following symptoms must be present in the late luteal phase of most cycles, with at least one symptom being from groups 1, 2, 3 or 4.

1. Clearly unstable mood (for example, sudden sadness).

2. Clear and persistent irritability or anger.

3. Clear anxiety, nervous tension, or feeling of being overwrought.

4. Clearly depressive mood, feeling of hopelessness, or reduction in self-esteem.

5. Reduced interest in activities such as work, family, friends or hobbies.

6. Rapid tiring and clear lack of energy.

7. Subjective feeling of not being able to concentrate.

8. Clear change in eating behaviour, such as increased appetite or craving for sweet foods.

9. Sleep disorders such as too much sleep or sleeplessness.

10. Other physical symptoms such as tender breasts, feeling of bloating, headache, joint or muscle pain, weight gain.

C: The symptoms are such that they are invariably noticeable and create difficulties in the normal course of daily life.

D: The symptoms are not merely an aggravated expression of the symptoms of other diseases such as depression.

Answer A3

Perhaps one of the most important things is to provide support and reassurance for her, explain that she is not alone or at all mad. You could also give her information leaflets and addresses of the support groups.

Life-style changes may be of benefit, such as increasing exercise and trying to reduce stress pre-menstrually. Maintaining blood sugar levels and switching to a 3-hourly starch diet has been shown to help some women.

The currently available non-hormonal pharmacological methods of treatment include evening primrose oil, containing gamolenic acid. This comes from the belief that PMS sufferers may be deficient in essential fatty acids and/or prostaglandin E1 that leads to higher sensitivity to normal physiological events in the ovarian cycle. In some studies, evening primrose oil and efemast (gamolenic acid 40 and 80 mg) have been shown to be superior to placebo in reducing symptoms, especially breast tenderness.

Pyridoxine (vitamin B_6) has been used effectively in some women. The rationale for its use is that high estrogen concentrations could cause a deficiency in pyridoxine, which could alter local dopamine and serotonin release and function. Studies have suggested that it can relieve depression in several conditions, especially those associated with high dose combined oral contraceptive pills. A meta-analysis concluded that there was some evidence to suggest pyridoxine (100 mg per day) was superior to placebo in relieving some of the symptoms of PMS, especially depression.

The fruits of agnus castus contain a mixture of iridoids and flavonoids, and some compounds similar to sex hormones. The effects of agnus castus are supposed to be similar to those of the corpus luteum. The mode of action may also be related to the stress-induced prolactin production modulated by dopamine. The extracts of these fruits have been proven to be beneficial in the treatment of the syndrome, with a 50% improvement in symptoms, high acceptance and low side effects.

Magnesium and calcium supplements (cofactors in the conversion of tryptophan and serotonin) have been shown to be useful. Similarly, antidepressants like the serotonin reuptake inhibitors (fluoxetine) have been shown to be useful, although it is sometimes difficult to explain to the patient that we are treating PMS not depression. However, there is no firm evidence of the efficacy of these medications.

Diuretics may be useful when the bloatedness is associated with weight gain. Spironolactone has been shown in one small study to improve mood.

Bromocriptine reduces dopamine levels and may be beneficial in reducing cyclical breast pain, and possibly some other symptoms of PMS, but further trials are needed.

Prostaglandin synthase inhibitors, especially mefenamic acid have been shown to be effective in controlling symptoms.

Danazol suppresses gonadotrophin secretion and thereby prevents ovarian function, but it has unacceptable side effects for many women. It would not be useful in this woman because it is contraindicated with a history of thromboembolism. This would also apply to estrogens, which some studies have shown can be beneficial in treating PMS. Although progestogens could be given alone, their validity in treating PMS is doubtful.

GnRH analogues may be useful to suppress gonadotrophin release, but can only be administered alone (without add-back HRT) for a maximum of 6 months. They may be useful prior to considering surgery so that Mrs Handcox would know what to experience after a hysterectomy.

Therefore, in view of the fact that Mrs Handcox's main complaints are breast tenderness, bloating and headaches, along with her perceived heavy periods, I would suggest she initially try mefenamic acid in combination with oil of evening primrose. This might help with her headaches, menorrhagia and breast tenderness.

Answer A4

The standard surgical management of PMS is to perform a hysterectomy with bilateral salpingo-oophorectomy. Most of these are done abdominally. The risks with this operation are significantly increased when compared with bilateral oophorectomy alone. However, a hysterectomy with bilateral salpingo-oophorectomy is chosen in order to prevent the development of endometrial cancer due to postoperative HRT (unopposed oestrogens).

In this woman's case, there may be some concerns about the use of oestrogens in view of the fact that she had a spontaneous DVT at the age of 22. It would be useful to find out if this was proven, was associated with any event (e.g. pregnancy, a broken leg), and what the family history was with relation to venous thromboembolism. You could also perform a thrombophilia screen on her.

It would be useful to try her with GnRH analogues in order to see whether 'medical castration' causes all of her symptoms to disappear.

Further reading

Baker PN, Fay TN, Hammond RH (1998) *Obstetrics and Gynaecology: cases, questions and commentaries*, pp. 175–178. WB Saunders Company, London.
(1992) Managing the premenstrual syndrome. *Drugs Therapeut. Bull.* **30**: 69–72.
O'Brien PMS, Chenoy R (1997) Premenstrual syndrome. In: Shaw RW, Soutter WP, Stanton SL (eds), *Gynaecology*, 2nd edn, pp. 359–371.
O'Brien PMS, Abukhalil IEH, Henshaw C (1995) Premenstrual syndrome. Curr. Obstet. Gynaecol. **5**: 30–35.
Schellenberg R (2001) Treatment for the premenstrual syndrome with agnus castus fruit extract: prospective, randomised, placebo controlled study. *Br. Med. J.* **322**: 134–137
Slade R et al. (1998) Premenstrual Syndrome. Key Topics in Obstetrics and Gynaecology, pp. 111–113. BIOS Scientific Publishers Ltd, Oxford.
Wyatt KM, Dimmock PW, Jones PW, O'Brien PMS (1999) Efficacy of vitamin B-6 in the treatment of premenstrual syndrome: systematic review. *Br. Med. J.* **318**: 1375–1381.

CIRCUIT 3

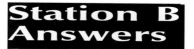

Station B Answers

Answer B1

Medical audit is the 'systematic and critical analysis of the quality of medical care, including the procedures used for diagnosis and treatment, the use of resources and the resulting outcome for the patient'.

An audit cycle is the sequence of events that starts from selection of a topic, then goes through adopting a standard, performing the audit, comparing the result with the standard, implementing change and repeating the audit until the standard is achieved.

Medical audit is the 'systematic and critical analysis of the quality of medical care carried out by doctors looking at the things that doctors do'. Clinical audit is the 'systematic and critical analysis carried out by all health professionals, including doctors when working with other health professionals, looking at the things that they do together.' Clinical audit can include lay people and is preferred to medical audit.

Structure is defined as: 'the availability and organization of the resources (e.g. staff and equipment) required for the delivery of a service.'

Process refers to: 'the way the patient is received and managed by the service from the time of referral until the time of discharge.'

Outcome means: 'the results of clinical intervention.'

Answer B2

The start of the audit cycle begins with selecting a topic, in this case the outcome following induction of labour. Second, a clear standard needs to be adopted; this can either be from National Guidelines and standards, or local ones. Third, the indicators to be measured are to be defined. Fourth, a target is to be set. Finally, the monitoring method is to be clearly defined. This must contain the following components:

- the method of data collection;
- the person responsible for the audit;
- the frequency with which the audit should be repeated.

We need to begin by defining induction of labour. Induction of labour is the artificial initiation of uterine contractions, prior to their spontaneous onset,

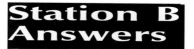

leading to progressive dilatation and effacement of the cervix and delivery of the baby. The question asks about an audit to investigate the outcomes following induction of labour, but does not distinguish between the reasons for induction of labour (which can be numerous).

To look at all the cases of induction of labour would include multiparous women and primiparous women, those pre-term (for instance with PET) and those post-term, those with normal babies and those with abnormal or dead babies, all where the outcomes may be expected to be different.

The RCOG recommends prostaglandins to initiate labour in primiparous women with an unripe cervix. This is an auditable standard – all women undergoing induction of labour with an unripe cervix should be given prostaglandins. Written guidelines are available and can be audited against, to see if these were adhered to or not.

The RCOG recommends induction of labour at 41 weeks and 4 days, or increased surveillance. This again is an auditable standard, and we can look to see at what point women in our hospital were induced, and the perinatal mortality rates associated with induction or surveillance. The RCOG has published guidelines on induction of labour.

We need to know about the indication for induction, methods used (including things like previous membrane sweeping, which should reduce the incidence of formal induction) and outcomes (failure rates, method of delivery and neonatal outcome).

The audit could either be retrospective or prospective. Most are retrospective (looking back) and it is following their results that practice is altered before a prospective audit is carried out. We also need to set time limits – those looked at and when to re-audit. The easiest way to collect data is to use a proforma, illustrated below, with the data being entered into a database for analysis. A proforma ensures that similar data are collected for each patient from each set of notes, and helps to record the information accurately and remove bias.

There is no agreement on the actual rate for induction of labour, but rates between 10 and 25% are common. Failure rates with prostaglandins are reported as being 3%.

Proforma for Induction of Labour

Name
Unit number
Date of birth
Age
Parity
  Details:

Reason for induction: Post-mature
                                    PET   Diabetic   Other maternal condition
                                    Twins   IUGR   Other fetal condition
                                    Fetal abnormality   FDIU
                                    Maternal request
Gestation when induction commenced:
Gestation determined by: LMP   Early scan   Late scan

Decision for induction: Midwife / SHO / SpR / Staff Grade / Consultant

Time of initial induction:
Method of induction: Sweep   PGs   Oxytocin   Amniotomy

Type and doses of PGs used:

Bishop's score at induction:

Date and time of delivery:

Method of delivery: Normal   Instrumental   CS
Reason for instrumental / CS:

Details of baby: Weight   Sex
                              Apgar scores
                              Other problems / abnormalities
Comments:

Answer B3

The induction rate overall is possibly a little high, but acceptable.

The two main reasons for performing inductions are post maturity and maternal request. Evidence suggests there is no benefit in inducing before 41 weeks, so 80 of these inductions may be unnecessary. There is also a high level of 'social inductions' for maternal request and no medical reason.

It is recommended that consultants are involved in the decision to undertake induction of labour, but this seems to be quite uncommon here. The majority of the decisions are made by the Staff Grades and SpRs. Some of these decisions may be questionable, and more consultant involvement is recommended.

There is a very high Caesarean section rate; most of these are attributed to failed induction. This again highlights the importance of case selection. It might be reduced if the time of induction for post maturity was agreed as being 41 weeks and maternal requests were limited, and all were fully discussed and made by a consultant.

The high failure rate may be reflected by the high level of use of prostaglandins, amniotomy and oxytocin – perhaps in many women with initially unfavourable Bishop's scores. Further breakdown of this would be useful. Amniotomy and oxytocin alone are not recommended as useful induction agents and the reasons for their use should be clarified.

Recommendations should be made, such as:

- no routine induction of labour for post-maturity before 41 completed weeks;

- no routine induction of labour for maternal request;

- the decision to induce should be made by a consultant;

- membrane sweeping is to be encouraged;

- amniotomy and oxytocin should not be used alone to induce labour.

The audit needs repeating after 12 months.

Answer B4

Some of the benefits of audit are:

- it provides evidence of patient care and improves the standard of care;

- it provides evidence to challenge or convince purchasers;

- it improves doctors' awareness of patients' views on the results of interventions;

- it is an excellent way of continuing education;

- it introduces changes in clinical practice;

- it helps in solving clinical or organizational problems;

- it helps in resolution of conflicts;

- it helps in getting approval of training programmes;

- it eliminates 'shroud waving';

- it improves job satisfaction;

- it helps in removing boundaries between GPs and hospital doctors and between different professional groups within the hospital.

The essential difference is that research determines what constitutes good care, whereas audit determines whether good care is being practised. While audit sets a standard to achieve, research determines what that standard should be. In audit there is a set target, whereas in research there is no pre-set target to reach.

Further reading

Chapple J (1995) Audit in obstetrics. In: Bonnar J (ed.), *Recent Advances in Obstetrics and Gynaecology,* No. 19, pp. 91–107. Churchill Livingstone, Edinburgh.

De Lacey G (1992) What is audit? Why should we be doing it? *Hospital Update* 458–466.
Enkin M, Keirse MJNC, Neilson J *et al.* (2000) *A Guide to Effective Care in Pregnancy and Childbirth,* 3rd edn, pp. 234–239 and 383–395. Oxford University Press, Oxford.
Royal College of Obstetricians and Gynaecologists (1997) Effective procedures in maternity care suitable for audit. Royal College of Obstetricians and Gynaecologists, London.
Royal College of Obstetricians and Gynaecologists (1998) Induction of labour. Guideline No. 16. Royal College of Obstetricians and Gynaecologists, London.

CIRCUIT 3

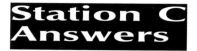

Answer C2: continue as a role play

I can confirm that you are about 8 weeks pregnant and would be happy to perform the termination for you.

What does the operation involve?

You would be admitted as a day case, which means that you would be in hospital hopefully for just a day. Before we do the operation we need to take some blood to test from you. On the day of the operation you must have nothing to eat or drink for at least 6 hours before. When you come in you will have a tablet inserted into your vagina at least an hour before the operation. This will cause the neck of the womb to soften up. It means that there are less likely to be complications with the operation, but it may make you feel a little sick and can cause you to start bleeding and get some crampy pains before the operation starts.

You will be put to sleep and the operation will take about 5 minutes to perform. We open up the neck of the womb and remove everything that is in there. You should be able to go home later that day and will normally bleed and get a few pains for several days.

You told me that I should tell my parents in case of complications – what did you mean by that?

There is a chance of you developing an infection after the operation. This is normally in the womb, but rarely could affect the tubes leading to their blockage. The rate of infection is about 2–5% after a surgical termination. To try and reduce this we can look for the infection beforehand by taking swabs or give you antibiotics that you must take for a full week afterwards.

Rarely, when we do the operation we can actually make a hole in the womb. If we do that you could bleed heavily or we could accidentally damage other things inside your tummy. We may need to look inside your tummy with a camera and there is a risk that we would need to make a big cut in your tummy and you would have to stay in hospital for days. You can also bleed from the neck of the womb or from inside the womb itself. Some people (1 in 200) bleed so much that they require a blood transfusion afterwards.

There is also a small risk that we do not completely empty your womb out and you could continue to bleed after the operation. Finally, some people can have problems with the general anaesthetic.

You make it sound awful – are there any other ways?

Yes, we can give you tablets to try and make you miscarry.

What are the risks with that?

There is still a risk of infection but it is much smaller (1–2% after medical termination). The other advantages are that it avoids the risks of damage to the womb and neck of the womb, and you don't need a general anaesthetic. You can still bleed afterwards and there is actually a slightly higher chance of requiring a blood transfusion (0.85%).

The big disadvantage is that it involves more visits to the hospital and there is a slightly higher chance of it not working (5%). If this is the case you would still need the operation.

Could I have the tablet termination today, because if I didn't have the anaesthetic I wouldn't need to tell my parents?

You can have the medical termination, because it can be done up to 9 weeks (63 days), but I would still recommend that you tell your parents. We can't do it today so you will need to come back to the hospital to take one tablet of a medicine called mifepristone (200 mg). We will keep an eye on you for a couple of hours before you can go home. You will then need to come back to the hospital 2 days (48 hours) after the first tablet for another medicine. During these 2 days you might have period-like pains or bleed, you might even miscarry at home (65%). If the bleeding is bad, or you get bad tummy pains you should come back to the hospital.

If the first tablet has not worked by itself, it makes the womb more likely to contract when we give you a different medicine called Misoprostol. This can be taken as a tablet or put inside your vagina. We prefer to put it into your vagina because this way it is less likely to give you side effects like diarrhoea. You may need more than one dose, but will stay in the hospital until the termination is complete.

Answer C3

The first thing I would do is explain to Debbie that her womb feels much bigger than it should be and we need to get a scan done to confirm exactly how many weeks pregnant she is and to see how many babies are there.

If the scan confirmed that she was 22 weeks pregnant with one baby, I would explain the options to her. First, she could continue with the pregnancy and keep the baby. If this was not an option she could consider adoption. Finally, some units might still be prepared to offer her a prostaglandin termination. I would need to find out which of the local units, if any, would consider this. There is also the possibility of sending her to a centre outside the area that might be willing to perform terminations up to 24 weeks. If this was to be the case I would discuss the fact that the fetus should be killed before the termination takes place.

Answer C4

I would tell her that her womb felt much smaller than it should be for someone who is 8 weeks pregnant. I would arrange an ultrasound scan of her uterus and ovaries to look for evidence of a miscarriage or an ectopic pregnancy and would check a serum βhCG to see if she had ever been pregnant.

Answer C5

I would agree to the termination under clause C of the Abortion Act, in that to continue the pregnancy is a greater danger to her health than if the pregnancy was terminated.

Answer C6

Debbie is only 15 years old so this man has had sex with her illegally. He is also her father, who is clearly abusing her. I would ask to see Debbie again and try to talk to her about this.

Fearing for Debbie's welfare I would contact social services. I would also ask advice from my senior colleagues and possibly discuss it with my defence union. The police should be informed even though it might be breaching patient confidentiality.

Further reading

Guillebaud J (1995) *Contraception Today*. Martin Dunitz Ltd, London.

Henshaw RC, Templeton AA (1993) Antiprogesterones. In: Studd J (ed.), *Progress in Obstetrics and Gynaecology*, Vol 10, pp. 259–280. Churchill Livingstone, Edinburgh.

Age of consent 16 years and contraceptive advice to under 16 years age group – The UK Memorandum of Guidance (DHSS HC(FP)86) (issued after the Gillick case).

Slade R *et al.* (1998) Therapeutic abortion. Key Topics in Obstetrics and Gynaecology, pp. 132–134.

CIRCUIT 3

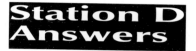

Answer D1

General impressions
The first thing to comment on is that it is encouraging that an information leaflet has been written, but it is dreadful.

The picture on the front cover is inappropriate, and although it is a cartoon, it seems to be a little threatening.

This leaflet uses many medical terms that are not simplified or explained, and many people would not understand it. General terms should be used so that people can understand them. If medical phrases are used they need an explanation. Overall, the leaflet is not reassuring, and is likely to generate more anxiety than if no information was sent at all. The word 'cancer' is used on several occasions – this should only be used in a positive way, such as 'unlikely to find cancer'.

The smear test
This is very badly written. The term 'cytological screening test' should be replaced by the word 'smear'. Patients do not need to know about 'exfoliated squamous epithelial cells', 'ectocervix' and the 'glandular cells from your endocervix'. Similarly, the terms 'mitotic activity', 'nuclear to cytoplasm ratios', 'mild dyskaryosis', 'micro-invasive cancer' are too medical and unnecessary. The paragraph could perhaps read:

'When a smear is taken the microscope doctors look for the cells that are shed from the outside of the neck of the womb and those at the entrance to the birth canal. They look for those that are normal and those that are not normal. It is the cells that are not normal that we are interested in.'

A diagram would be useful here.

'The test may also have revealed that you are infected with the wart virus (human papilloma virus), which may be contributing to the abnormalities.' This suggests that the woman may be infected with the wart virus. Many people associate this with sexually transmitted infections and genital warts – it is misleading and could cause anxiety.

Your first visit to the colposcopy clinic
This begins with a sentence that makes people think that smears are inaccurate and therefore questions the reason why they are done. It then continues to

explain what is a colposcopy. I think the sentence is an acceptable one, but 'large microscope' conjures up the wrong image.

It is important to inform the patients that the hospital is a teaching hospital, but it makes it sound like there are going to be lots of people in the room. If the patient does not want the observers in the room, it is up to them to ask for the observers to leave. The words 'forced to leave' imply that the patients are wrong and should not ask for this. This should be the other way around. The doctor should ask the patient if it is acceptable to them to have observers, and if they agree then only one or two observers should be admitted.

The phrase, 'When you come to the clinic you will be met by a doctor who might be strange to you', suggests that the doctor may be odd – not the sort of thing to reassure you. It is better practice to introduce yourself to the patient first and talk to them before they change into a gown, so that they feel vulnerable for the shortest period of time. Every time the doctor is mentioned it is always as 'he', which may not be the case, and could upset some women.

It is important to mention about asking questions, but again medical terms like 'parity' are used. It is again threatening and unnecessary to mention sexually transmitted diseases.

The description of the colposcopy couch makes it seem like a torture chamber – strapping legs in and having their 'innermost parts examined'.

The phrase, 'It is very important to be relaxed during the entire procedure otherwise it will hurt more', implies that colposcopy always hurts and will generate anxiety.

When the leaflet goes on to explain about the actual procedure it again mentions 'signs of cancer or pre-cancer'. This makes it seem like these changes are common; normality is not mentioned and anxiety will increase.

'He will then paint the neck of the womb with different solutions. The first one is an acid ....' People generally associate acid with burns, and would expect this to hurt. The next lines about the iodine make it sound like the doctor is incompetent and needs this second test to make sure he has not missed anything.

Again medical terms are used: 'histopathologists' and 'cytological findings'. These could be replaced with 'microscope doctors' and 'smear report'. The way that the biopsy is taken sounds horrendous with 'sharp pincers that cut into the cervix'. It would be better to talk about taking small pinches of the skin. Again the connotations are pain – 'it doesn't normally hurt very much'. It would be better to say that it is normally painless.

The fact that bleeding is mentioned is acceptable, but it is probably unnecessary to mention 'bleeding heavily'. Complications should be mentioned and, if possible, clarified for their occurrence and treatment. 'Silver nitrate' is a medical term that needs explanation.

Your second visit to the clinic

This implies that most people will come back for a further visit, and will probably make people feel worried. Again, medical terms are used such as 'cytologists' and 'histopathologists', instead of simple terms like 'microscope doctors' and 'smear results'.

The phrase, 'Depending on what grade of CIN or cancer they may show will determine how we subsequently manage you' makes you think that all results will show abnormalities, and for the first time introduces the term CIN without clarification or explanation of the abbreviation. Once more, it mentions cancer unnecessarily, and then goes on to talk about hysterectomies. Although this is probably written for comfort, it is not needed in an information leaflet about colposcopy. It would scare the majority of women, especially when it talks of radiotherapy to try and effect a cure.

The line 'If the biopsy shows CIN 2 or 3 you will require further treatment with a LLETZ' means absolutely nothing to a lay person. The terms CIN 2 and 3 have not been explained, nor has the full definition of LLETZ been described. Moreover, the way that a LLETZ is described as an 'electric current through a wire moving across your cervix whilst you are awake' sounds very unpleasant, and would not decrease anxiety levels. Similarly, with the description of the cone biopsy.

We now finally see what the abbreviation LLETZ stands for, but there is no mention of what this actually means. The fact that local anaesthetic is used should be comforting, but not so. It mentions injection of 'lots of local anaesthetic through many needle-pricks', which suggests a painful and complex procedure involving lots of injections. You would hope that once this is done there is no feeling, but the reader is still not consoled – 'Usually, although not always . . . . you will not feel any pain.'

The connection to the 'electricity generating machine' again suggests that this is a vehicle of torture; it sounds like the woman is being connected to the electric chair. Again, there are mentions of burns and the smell of burning, making the process sound horrendous and very unpleasant.

The complications are again mentioned, but the haemorrhage is perhaps too detailed and threatening with the mention of blood transfusions and return to theatre. There is no mention of how long intercourse should be avoided and tampons used.

The sentence about CIN 1 is not as comforting as it is designed to be, talking about progression to 'more invasive disease' and the association with 'more invasive disease in the surrounding area'. This needs clarifying, simplifying and made to sound less worrying.

CIRCUIT 3

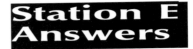

Answer E1

With regard to the documents

In this particular case the woman had an unplanned pregnancy and was consequently a late booker. She requested a termination, but by then she was over 18 weeks and this service was not offered locally. She had made an attempt at contraception in the form of Depo-Provera, but had not reattended for her repeat injection 3 months beforehand. Whether one would have been sufficient given her size is unlikely. With regard to future contraception and her request for sterilization, I would not be keen to support this for two reasons. First, her age (<25) and second, because her daughter is showing signs of developmental delay. If there were further problems with her daughter she may wish to have another child.

She is a poorly controlled insulin-dependent diabetic who was not well controlled pre-pregnancy, as seen by her elevated HbA_1C level in the booking letter. She is also obese for her height. The growth scans would also suggest poor control during her pregnancy, and the discharge summary reiterates this.

The pregnancy had also been complicated by a previous admission with pre-term labour, possibly because of the size of the baby.

The partogram reveals a normal spontaneous labour at 34 weeks. The fetal heart rate remained satisfactory and the liquor was clear throughout – nothing to suggest fetal distress. The membranes appeared to have ruptured spontaneously at 2 cm. Following rupture of the membranes, the contractions appear to have become a little stronger initially. She required pethidine in labour on two occasions, and following its administration her blood pressure and pulse dropped as normal. She did not appear to have required any stronger analgesia or the use of syntocinon.

Although she made slow progress over the first 5 hours, there was descent of the head, and once she was in established labour she progressed reasonably well. There is nothing to suggest an obstructed labour (contractions diminishing, no descent of fetal head, need for syntocinon, moulding, etc.) or the imminent shoulder dystocia.

We have not been given the details of why she required a forceps delivery, but the discharge summary clearly states that there was a shoulder dystocia and her episiotomy was extended giving rise to a third degree tear. The obstetrician should have been aware that this was likely to occur due to her size and the weight of her son born previously.

The planned hospital follow-up is appropriate after her tear; the choice of codeine as an analgesic and in combination with ferrous sulfate would be likely to cause constipation, which is not ideal.

Her daughter Kylie had some predicted problems, such as the hypoglycaemia and RDS, appropriate for a premature macrosomic baby. However, the birth trauma that resulted in fractures and brachial plexus injury would reiterate that this was a severe shoulder dystocia.

The record keeping in Document 6 is appalling. Whenever an instrumental delivery is performed abdominal palpation should be recorded before the vaginal examination findings. The vaginal findings should include the station and a forceps should not be attempted until the position is known. There is no mention of the type of forceps and whether or not they were easily applied, and how easy it was to deliver the head. There is no mention of the colour of the liquor or strength and frequency of contractions. There is no mention of any analgesia used, and abbreviations should only be recorded where they are standard. We presume that RMLE means right mediolateral episiotomy, but this is not a standard abbreviation (like CTG/VE which are acceptable).

Once a shoulder dystocia is diagnosed there is no mention as to what procedures were undertaken to try and deliver the shoulders before the registrar arrived. Each entry should be signed, and if it is the first entry the name and position of the doctor should be written legibly underneath.

Once the registrar arrived he obviously managed to deliver the baby, but has not recorded which manoeuvres he performed and in what order to achieve the delivery. Ideally, the times should be recorded for each different procedure. He has recorded '? Fracture' – but of what? He has recorded that there is a third degree tear, but has not defined this further. Third degree tears should ideally be repaired in theatre with effective analgesia, which is normally not local anaesthetic. The type of suture material and method of repair must also be documented.

There is no mention of the third stage and whether the placenta looked normal and complete. There is no record of the condition of the infant at birth. There is nothing relating to a rectal or vaginal examination at the end of the procedure, and that the swabs and instruments were checked and correct.

With regard to the allegations
1. The discharge summary implies that Evelyn had repeated visits to the clinic and was seen with a diabetologist each week. Although there is no documentation that states the risks have been discussed this is more than likely to have occurred.
2. The scans suggested that Kylie was a large baby, but Evelyn had previously delivered a 4.1 kg baby, she was admitted in spontaneous labour and did not have a particularly long labour. There was nothing to suggest the need for a caesarean section.
3. This is likely to be the case.
4. There is no guarantee that a caesarean would have protected against developmental delay.

5. The risks of developing stress incontinence are increased following traumatic vaginal deliveries and vaginal delivery of large babies. A caesarean may not have prevented this from occurring because of the fact that she had previously had a large baby. Also, there are some women who develop stress incontinence without ever having had a normal vaginal delivery.

The left arm injury is a direct result of birth trauma, but when clavicles are broken the situation is desperate. The child is probably lucky to be alive.

Answer E2

Clinical risk management (CRM) identifies procedures that may carry actual or legal hazards and minimizes them through formal safeguards and protocols. The RCOG defines CRM as:

> 'Methods for the early identification of adverse events, using either staff reports or systematic screening of records. This should be followed by creation of a database to identify common patterns and develop a system of accountability to prevent future incidents'.

Initially it was thought to be a means of controlling litigation, but became a way to consider strategies to reduce harm. The narrow view of CRM is negative and defensive, aimed primarily to protect hospitals from claims without any regard to the reasons for claims or to patient well being. On the positive side, CRM is fundamentally an approach to improving patient care with an emphasis on patients who are actually harmed or disturbed by their treatment. Complaints and litigation are part of this procedure. It is designed to be a reflective practice, rather than one based on ways to reduce litigation. CRM is now a part of clinical governance.

Answer E3

Clinical governance is part of day-to-day working practice in the NHS today. Clinical risk management is an integral part of clinical governance. The Commission for Health Improvement (CHI) carries overall responsibility to ensure that NHS trusts undertake clinical governance, and the Clinical Negligence Scheme for Trusts (CNST) carries similar responsibilities relating specifically to clinical risk management. Each hospital has CNST standards and these relate to the amount of money that the trust pays to protect itself against litigation claims.

Medicolegal claims are a major problem in the National Health Service. These have increased from £53 million in 1990/1991 to £125 million in 1994. The current cost is £100–£150 million per year, which constitutes 0.5% of the NHS budget. It looks negligible, but studies have shown that litigation underestimates the incidence of adverse events. The Harvard Study in 1989 demonstrated that the number of adverse events was seven-times that of claims and 14-times that of paid claims. In 1975–1978 the Californian Study showed that 1 in 10 patients with an injury due to error filed for malpractice, of which 40% were compensated. This means that 1 in 25 injuries due to probable negligence resulted in compensation.

The USA has been a prime mover in CRM, because the malpractice costs to healthcare were over $1 billion in 1985 and are rising. Adverse events happened in 370 per 10 000 admissions (4%). Of these 4%, 14% died (0.56% of all admissions), 7% suffered permanent disability (0.28% of all admissions) and 70% suffered temporary disability (2.8% of all admissions). If these statistics are transferred to England for annual admissions of 8 000 000, this implies 320 000 adverse events resulting in 40 000 deaths and 20 000 permanent disabilities per year. In an average district general hospital in England with 50 000 admissions per year, this implies 1850 adverse events, resulting in 75 deaths and 37 permanent disabilities annually.

The NHS executive has launched a risk management campaign to combat increasing litigation and claims and prevent them from crippling the National Health Service. Obstetrics and gynaecology is a high-risk speciality and accounted for the second largest (25%) settlement by the Medical Defence Union between August and October 1994. The usual obstetric causes of negligence were retained swabs or instruments (29%), operative injuries (18.3%), perinatal death (17.2%), brain-damaged babies (9.7%), antenatal problems (5.4%), perineal damage (4.3%) and others (16.1%). Common problems in gynaecology were failure to obtain informed consent, failure to inform the patient of potential risks and consequences of operations, delayed diagnosis of ectopic pregnancy, operative injuries, retained swabs and instruments, lack of supervision during operative procedures, perforation of the uterus, etc. CRM is expected to improve the standard of patient care and reduce malpractice.

Answer E4

The four fundamental principles of CRM are risk identification, analysis, control and funding. The starting point is to recognise what could go wrong, and what did go wrong. This requires the definition of clinical incidents that could give rise to significant harm to the patient. Once these have been identified, we need to analyze how often they are likely to occur. The last step is to plan how to eliminate the risk. The same steps are followed to find the causative factors, the severity of the effect, the cost and, finally, how to avoid the adverse event.

CRM cannot eliminate litigation, but it can certainly reduce the number of adverse incidents giving rise to litigation by rectifying human factors responsible for adverse clinical events.

The important aspects of clinical practice that could reduce malpractice are conscientious practice, good communication, careful and complete record keeping, taking informed consent, proper delegation and clinical risk management.

Answer E5

These are of two types: error and violation. Errors may be subdivided into slips, lapses, trips or fumbles, which are failures or deviations that occur at the level of the execution of the action. Slips and lapses are unintended actions despite an adequate plan. Slips occur due to attention failures and lapses are memory failures.

Mistakes are rule-based or knowledge-based. Rule-based mistakes may occur due to a bad rule or non-application of a good rule. Knowledge-based mistakes may occur due to bias or mindset, resulting in planning or problem-solving failures. Mistakes are failures of intention, when the action may go entirely as planned, but the plan is inadequate to achieve the outcome.

Violation may occur due to routine corner cutting, personal 'kicks' or necessity when it is the only available option.

Further reading

Doherty R, James CE (1994) Malpractice in obstetrics and gynaecology. In: Bonnar J (ed.), *Recent Advances in Obstetrics and Gynaecology,* No. 18, pp. 91–106. Churchill Livingstone, Edinburgh.

Irvine LM (1996) Practical risk management advice on the labour ward. In: Studd J (ed.), *Progress in Obstetrics and Gynaecology,* Vol. 12, pp. 59–65. Churchill Livingstone, Edinburgh.

RCOG (2001) Clinical Risk Management for Obstetricians and Gynaecologists. RCOG Clinical Governance Advice No. 2. Royal College of Obstetricians and Gynaecologists, London.

CIRCUIT 3

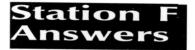

Answer F1

The first thing to do is make sure there is adequate help available. The consultant on call should be informed and a paediatrician should be present at the birth. It is also sensible to make the on-call theatre staff and anaesthetist aware of the problem.

Having confirmed that this was a shoulder dystocia, I would then take the legs out of the lithotomy position and perform the McRoberts manoeuvre by flexing the maternal thighs up onto the maternal abdomen, they should also be abducted and externally rotated. This simulates the advantages of a squatting position, increasing the pelvic inlet diameter. The McRoberts manoeuvre also corrects the lumbosacral lordosis, removing the sacral promontory as a potential obstruction. At the same time, this manoeuvre flexes the fetal spine, and often pushes the posterior shoulder over the sacral promontory, allowing it to descend into the hollow of the sacrum. The direction of maternal force in this position is perpendicular to the plane of the inlet, and delivery should occur with normal traction in under a minute.

Although an episiotomy has already been performed it may be necessary to extend it, especially if you think you will be unable to readily access the vagina and fetus to perform rotational manoeuvres if necessary.

While exerting normal traction on the baby, I would ask one of the midwives present to press down suprapubically on the anterior shoulder, forcing it anterior with regards to the fetal trunk. She should be holding her hands as if performing cardiac massage, with her palm flat. This should help to adduct the shoulders and reduce the bisacromial diameter. This should be attempted for no longer than 1 minute. Initially, the pressure can be continuous, but if delivery is not accomplished, a rocking motion is advocated to dislodge the shoulder from behind the pubic symphysis. If this fails, the next procedure should be immediately attempted.

Internal manual pressure should then be applied for the next 30 seconds. This involves adduction of the most accessible fetal shoulder while traction is continued. Initially, this is done using the internal hand behind the maternal symphysis pushing on the posterior aspect of the anterior shoulder of the baby to adduct the shoulder. The pressure on the posterior aspect of the anterior shoulder may be done simultaneously with pressure on the posterior clavicle, creating enough force to rotate the fetus into an oblique position.

If this is unsuccessful, the rotation should quickly be attempted in the opposite direction, the 'Woods Screw' manoeuvre. I would apply pressure to the posterior aspect of the posterior shoulder and attempt to rotate it into an oblique position. This should simultaneously dislodge the impacted anterior shoulder. If this fails, the manoeuvre is completed by continuing the rotation a full 180 degrees, so that the anterior shoulder becomes the posterior one. If rotating through 180 degrees, it will be necessary to change hands to complete the rotation. This should allow the delivery to occur.

If the shoulders were still stuck I would try and deliver the posterior arm. To do this, I would place my hand in the posterior aspect of the vagina in front of the baby. If the baby were facing left I would use my right hand, if it were facing right I would use my left. After identifying the posterior arm I would try to flex it at the shoulder and elbow in order to retrieve the hand or the forearm. The hand or forearm is then flexed across the face in an upward direction to deliver the arm. The anterior shoulder will normally follow.

This procedure is sometimes associated with fractures of the humerus or clavicles. If I thought that had occurred I would warn the parents, but tell them they usually heal well without any long-term sequelae. Each manoeuvre or procedure should be tried in rapid succession. It is pointless and dangerous to struggle with a single manoeuvre. Likewise, continued maternal pushing and traction are not helpful and may result in brachial plexus injuries.

If all of the above procedures have failed, cephalic replacement could be attempted, the 'Zavanelli manoeuvre', followed by a caesarean section. This involves flexion of the fetal head when it is in a direct occipital anterior position followed by cephalic replacement with continuous pressure on the fetal head until the section occurs. Tocolysis with nifedipine may be valuable in this situation. The other last-try technique is to perform a symphysiotomy. If this were attempted I would insert a metal catheter into the urethra to push it laterally. Having injected some local anaesthesia into the skin over the symphysis pubis I would take a scalpel and cut downwards. The disadvantages with this procedure are urinary tract damage and pelvic fractures.

Answer F2

I would begin by explaining that shoulder dystocia means that the shoulders fail to rotate and enter the pelvis once the baby's head has been delivered. Although a dystocia this bad is uncommon, it may affect up to 2% of vaginal deliveries to some degree. Unfortunately, it is a diagnosis made at the time and cannot be predicted.

I would explain to the parents that there are certain risk factors that increase the likelihood of this occurring, such as diabetes, obesity, a prolonged second stage, instrumental delivery, and large babies over 4 kg. She had these risk factors, but having an increased risk does not mean that a shoulder dystocia will occur. I would also point out that over 50% of cases occur in babies under 4 kg and 70% in women who appear to have been labouring normally. Hence, it is impossible to prevent shoulder dystocia.

Evelyn is diabetic, which increases the risk by more than 70%, but she had previously had an uneventful delivery of a baby over 4 kg and an elective section at 34 weeks would not have been recommended.

With regard to the actual delivery, I would explain that all the simple measures we tried to allow the shoulders to deliver had failed. It became necessary to try more traumatic manoeuvres to deliver the baby alive. It is recognized that fractures can and do occur, and although they may cause some pain and bruising – possibly contributing to the physiological jaundice – there are no long-term detrimental effects.

The baby sounds like it has an Erb's palsy. This is caused by excessive traction on the brachial plexus (C5, 6, 7). Treatment is support and physiotherapy, and recovery is variable depending on the amount of nerve trauma originally incurred.

Answer F3

The first thing would be to try to anticipate the problem before it occurs. This woman was a poorly controlled diabetic; she was obese and had previously given birth to a baby boy weighing in excess of 4 kg. The growth scans in this pregnancy had indicated another macrosomic baby. The higher risk from a shoulder dystocia should have been recognized and documented in the labour notes, and a senior obstetrician should have been present at the birth in anticipation.

To try to improve outcomes, different manoeuvres should not be tried for long periods of time and excessive force should be avoided. Pneumonics like 'HELPERR' (**Help**, **E**pisiotomy, **L**egs, **P**ressure, **E**nter vagina, **R**emove posterior arm, **R**oll patient) are useful to remember all the procedures, and the order in which to try them. Fire drills should occur regularly on labour ward. These should involve all staff and encourage logical practice. Mannequins are useful if available.

It is also essential to keep accurate and detailed records. Someone should document the times and the procedures attempted with their outcomes. Critical incidence forms should be completed for cases like this and the delivery reviewed by senior clinicians.

Further reading

Neil AMC, Thornton S (2000) Shoulder dystocia – Pace Review. *The Obstetrician and Gynaecologist* **2**(4): 45–47.
Pearson JF (1996) Shoulder dystocia. *Curr Obstet. Gynaecol.* **6**: 30–34.

CIRCUIT 3

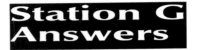

Answer G2

The semen analysis reveals a normal pH and volume. The sperm concentration is at the lower limit of normal, but both the motility and morphology are low. This should be repeated and a swim-up test performed to see if sufficient sperm could be recovered for assisted reproductive techniques.

Normal semen analysis (WHO, 1987):

Volume	$\geqslant 2$ ml
Sperm concentration	$\geqslant 20 \times 10^6$/ml
Motility	$\geqslant 50\%$ with forward progression
Morphology	$\geqslant 50\%$ with normal morphology
pH	7.2–7.8

The day 21 progesterone is normal, suggestive of ovulation, but without follicular tracking scans we can not exclude a LUF.

The laparoscopy has revealed two problems. The first, confirmed by the HSG is that there is cervical stenosis. The second is that there is endometriosis. It may be possible to try and bring her back at the time of a period to try and dilate the cervix, or to try and drill a hole with a laser. If this were not feasible then intrauterine insemination and embryo transfer would not be possible.

With regard to the endometriosis, there is no role for medical management, but there is some evidence to suggest that surgery improves fertility. I would recommend excision of the endometriosis laparoscopically, as this appears to be associated with lower rates of recurrence of the disease. However, although there is anecdotal evidence to say that surgical treatment for endometriosis improves IVF success rates, this has not been substantiated yet in large trials.

Overall, given the findings and assuming that his sperm count is satisfactory, the options available to them are GIFT or IVF with ZIFT (zygote intra-fallopian transfer). IVF is the more widely accepted treatment, but Mrs Beck would require a general anaesthetic to have the embryos replaced through her fallopian tubes if cervical access was impossible. It would be reasonable to bring her back when menstruating to see if it were feasible to cannulate her cervix with a fine embryo replacement catheter.

Answer G3

I would initially begin by explaining what is meant by IVF and explain the treatment cycle:

- down regulation with GnRH analogues;

- commencing stimulation with FSH;

- monitoring follicular development with scans and hormone analysis – estradiol levels;

- the egg recovery – transvaginally;

- the need for a sperm sample on the day of the recovery;

- the fertilization process;

- embryo replacement – maximum of 2 embryos;

- luteal phase support;

- freezing excess, but apparently normal embryos for future use.

Prior to IVF they would need blood tests to check their hepatitis and HIV status. If Vicky had previously not had her rubella and syphilis status checked these should also be checked.

The complications, success rates and failures need to be discussed:

- success rates – 20–30% reported per treatment cycle started;

- increased success with more embryos replaced, but higher multiple pregnancy rates;

- cycles abandoned if poor response;

- cycles abandoned if OHSS occurs.

The risks of OHSS need to be explained and the need for freezing all of the embryos if this occurs.

They need to be reassured that if a pregnancy occurs, the pregnancy does not appear to be at a higher risk of miscarrying, but there is an increased risk of ectopic pregnancy. Children born from IVF appear to be normal in all respects, but at present we do not know if second generation children will also be normal.

The IVF counselling should also make reference to the fact that in Great Britain IVF is licensed by the Human Fertilisation and Embryo Authority (HFEA), who make annual inspection visits, collate data and have records of all IVF treatments undertaken. The couple should inform the centre of the outcome of any pregnancies for this purpose. As part of this legislation in the Human Fertilisation and Embryo Act, the IVF centre has a responsibility to take into account the welfare of any child born by IVF. This may be relevant to the risk of triplets or if there is concern about the relationship of the potential parents, or because of severe medical or psychiatric complications.

The couple need to be informed that the child is legally their own, and any child can request information at the age of eighteen to see if they were conceived by IVF and donated sperm, oocytes or embryos.

They also need to be ensured of the confidentiality of the treatment and they need to consent to the disclosure of information about themselves to other parties not directly involved in the treatment (e.g. their GP).

Finally they should be offered counselling by a non-medical, trained counsellor at any point during their proposed treatment.

Further reading

Hunter DC (2001) The management of advanced-stage endometriosis in the treatment of infertility. *The Obstetrician and Gynaecologist* **3**(1): 4–7.

Jones WR (1995) Infertility. In: Whitfield CR (ed.), *Dewhurst's Textbook of Obstetrics and Gynaecology for Postgraduates*, 5th edn, pp. 551–561. Blackwell Scientific Publications, Oxford.

Read J (1995) Infertility counselling. In: Jacobs H (ed.), *Infertility*, 2nd edn, pp. 58–60. Reed Healthcare Communications, Surrey.

Slade R *et al.* (1998) Infertility. Key Topics in Obstetrics and Gynaecology, pp. 57–64. BIOS Scientific Publishers Ltd, Oxford.

Thompson W, Heasley RN (1992) Investigation of the infertile couple. In: Shaw RW, Soutter WP, Stanton SL (ed.), *Gynaecology*, pp. 219–229. Churchill Livingstone, Edinburgh.

Any paper by David Redwine is recommended reading.

CIRCUIT 3

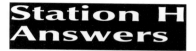

Answer H1

Initially, I would take a full history and examine her. From her history I would like to know more about her current problems and the amount of disturbance in her lifestyle they cause.

With regard to the stress incontinence, I would ask about what brings it on (laughing, sneezing, exercise, intercourse) and any factors that might make it worse, such as chronic cough and constipation. With regard to her urgency and urge incontinence, I would enquire about her voiding patterns and ask whether she has ever noticed pain or blood when passing urine. I would ascertain her drinking habits and drug intake. I would also enquire about neurological symptoms (like visual disturbance, problems walking) and backache. I would also ascertain any relevant medical and surgical problems and look for symptoms of prolapse and oestrogen deficiency.

I would then examine her thoroughly. It is important to exclude the presence of any abdominopelvic masses or ascites on abdominal palpation. If a neurological problem is suspected then the cranial nerves and sacral nerve roots S2, 3 and 4 should be examined, and nystagmus checked for. I would then perform a vaginal examination. A cystourethrocele can be diagnosed by vaginal examination. Any demonstrable stress incontinence, atrophic changes and tenderness over the urethra and bladder are also checked during the examination. The size of the uterus and any uterovaginal prolapse should be elucidated.

I would then explain to her that it sounds like she has both types of incontinence – stress and urge – and would define what we mean by each term. I would tell her that her symptoms might be caused by several factors, like prolapse of the bladder and urethra (cystourethrocele), weakness of the bladder neck (genuine stress incontinence, GSI) or an unstable bladder (detrusor instability, DI). I would inform her that we would need to undertake some further tests to tell us exactly what is going on, because the treatment of these problems is essentially different. Therefore, it is necessary to find the exact diagnosis before embarking on the treatment.

I would send a midstream specimen of urine for culture and sensitivity to exclude a urinary tract infection and to look for microscopic haematuria that might indicate bladder pathology. I would encourage her to keep a frequency-volume chart. I would refer her to the urodynamic clinic for a pad test, cystometry and uroflowmetry to get a diagnosis. I would also refer her to the physiotherapist to start pelvic floor exercises while she awaits the urodynamic studies. If atrophic changes were present I would advise her to use estrogen cream locally.

Answer H2

The commonest cause of urinary incontinence in women is GSI, and DI is the second most common cause. These two account for more than 90% of cases of female urinary incontinence.

Although 98% of women with GSI complain of stress incontinence, 25% of those with DI do also. Eighty-nine percent of women with DI and 37% of those with GSI complain of urge incontinence. It is also possible for the two to coexist – GSI is associated with DI in 25–30% of cases.

The clinical diagnosis does not correlate well with the urodynamic diagnosis – 'the bladder is an unreliable witness' (in studies done by Jarvis et al., only 68% of those with GSI and 51% of those with DI were correctly diagnosed by history). As their treatment differs, making an accurate initial diagnosis is very important.

The other advantage of urodynamics is that it allows the stability of the detrusor muscle to be assessed prior to surgery, and a baseline test is done prior to definitive treatment.

Dual channel subtraction cystometry is relatively cheap and a widely available technique that is highly likely to be informative. It enables detrusor instability to be elicited with low compliance during the filling phase, and when combined with the stress test (e.g. cough, heal rolling). It can effectively rule out or confirm GSI and/or DI.

Answer H3

A frequency-volume chart might suggest detrusor instability, but it cannot diagnose it. DI is suggested by observing frequent voiding of relatively small volumes of urine.

The best test to distinguish between the two types of incontinence is a filling cystometrogram. If this is not diagnostic of any pathology (as occurs in up to 8% of investigations) and the symptoms are strongly suggestive of DI, it should either be repeated or ambulatory urodynamics arranged. These will detect DI in up to 65% of patients where a cystometrogram was normal.

Answer H4

I would treat the DI first before embarking on any operative treatment for GSI. My reason for this is that the DI may persist or even worsen post-operatively causing further deterioration of the symptoms of incontinence, making it even more difficult to treat. Medical management of DI could be combined with pelvic floor exercises. This may result in an improvement in the mixed incontinence, potentially avoiding an operation altogether.

Answer H5

(This is the author's preferred method of treatment, it is not necessarily the right way. If you offer the more efficacious and effective [but difficult to gain access to] behavioural therapies, then that is fine. Most people would not recommend surgery as a first line.)

Detrusor instability can be very difficult to treat as it is usually a chronic condition with fixed voiding habits and behavioural patterns. The contribution of psychological factors is not clear, but women with high anxiety scores respond badly to medical treatments.

The first step is to explain the underlying problem and reassure the woman that it is common, affecting up to a quarter of women, and that we have ruled out any pathology as a cause of the problem. Women with mild symptoms may not require anything more than this simple reassurance, and advice on avoiding tea, coffee, alcohol and excessive fluid intake, and perhaps changing medications that promote urination (e.g. diuretics). There is a vast range of treatments available for women with severe symptoms, including drugs, behavioural therapy, maximal electrical stimulation, hypnosis and acupuncture and, finally, surgical procedures.

I would begin treatment with drugs, usually anticholinergics. They are generally cheap, easy to administer and you can treat more women per unit time than with behavioural approaches. Estrogens may help with some symptoms although there is no evidence to say that they are superior to placebo when treating genuine DI. In this particular case I would not recommend an anticholinergic drug because of her history of glaucoma.

Anticholinergic drugs are effective, but their use is limited by their systemic side effects, such as dry mouth, drowsiness, blurred vision, tachycardia, constipation and urinary retention. I would normally commence oxybutynin hydrochloride at a dose of 2.5 mg daily, gradually increasing it to 5 mg two to three times daily to improve the tolerance of the patient to the side effects. This approach is particularly useful in elderly women. It relieves symptoms in about 60% of cases. Dryness of mouth is the major side effect, occurring in up to 88% of patients. Tolterodine (2 mg twice a day) is a newer drug with fewer side effects. It is better tolerated, but does not appear to be as efficacious as oxybutynin. Propiverine also has calcium channel-blocking properties, and it may be superior to oxybutynin, although further studies are awaited. Propantheline is not popular because of its side effects, which are unacceptable to 1 in 5 women, and the requirement for higher dosages (30–60 mg daily). It is only indicated in adult enuresis (15–30 mg three times daily).

Tricyclic antidepressants (e.g. imipramine 50–150 mg nocte, amitriptyline 25–75 mg nocte) may be useful for patients with nocturia. 1-Desamino-8-D-arginine vasopressin (DDAVP) is a long acting analogue of vasopressin and reduces the urine production by 50% after a single dose of 20–40 mg. It is useful in enuresis and nocturia. It is safe for long-term use, but is contraindicated in women with cardiac disease, hypertension and epilepsy.

Behavioural therapy in the form of 'bladder drill', to mimic the learning process of infancy to consciously inhibit the voiding reflex, has been reported to establish continence in 84% of cases, and 76% of cases remain symptom free initially. The drawback is that it is time-consuming and requires an intelligent and highly motivated patient. The best chance of success seems to be with an inpatient admission. The high relapse rate of 40% after 3 years may precipitate a further admission to repeat the 'bladder drill'.

Other treatments, like maximal electrical stimulation, biofeedback, hypnosis, and acupuncture have been shown to be effective but are all very time-consuming.

With regard to surgery, there is no place for bladder transection, urethral dilatation, vaginal denervation or transvesical phenol injections. There are only two treatments currently advocated. Prolonged bladder distension needs adequate regional analgesia and the bladder should remain filled for 2 hours. The main problems with this are the risks of bladder rupture (8%) and overall poor improvement in fewer than 50% of patients. Augmentation 'clam' ileocystoplasty may have a place in some selected patients who have failed to respond to other measures and urinary diversion is the only alternative. The cure rate is about 90%, but voiding difficulties are common and may necessitate clean intermittent self-catheterization (CISC) in about 10%. Mucus secreted by the ileal mucosa may be troublesome, and there is a risk of adenocarcinoma developing in the ileal segment.

Answer H6

These include conservative and surgical treatments. Conservative measures are effective in 40–90% of cases. The available modalities are pelvic floor physiotherapy, electrical treatment, devices and medication. These have few complications and do not compromise future surgery. Improved success rates seem to occur if the physiotherapist is interested in these problems. Pelvic floor exercises without supervision may be counterproductive. Mechanical devices that insert into the urethra or vagina are now available and are effective in some women.

With regard to surgery, the operation performed should be aimed at the type of incontinence identified. There appear to be two things responsible for GSI: urethral hypermobility and intrinsic sphincter deficiency. Operations that reposition the bladder are successful in the treatment of urethral hypermobility. If there is intrinsic sphincter deficiency then peri-urethral bulking agents and semi-obstructive slings are useful.

The most effective procedures in terms of long-term cure rates are retropubic suspensions and slings. The most widely performed operation is the Burch colposuspension with a success rate of about 90% when done as a first procedure. In this procedure I would make a low transverse suprapubic skin incision and enter the retropubic space to identify the bladder neck. I would then insert two sutures of PDS (polyglycolic acid) into the paravaginal fascia on each side. The first I would place near to the bladder-neck, the second about 1 cm proximal to that. The sutures should then be inserted into the ipsilateral ileopectineal ligament. The sutures are then tied to elevate the vagina, and they are tied lax. The complications associated with this are haemorrhage, injury to the bladder or ureter, kinking of the ureter, voiding difficulties (25%), detrusor instability (18.5%), enterocele (18%), dyspareunia and recurrence. Colposuspension can also be done laparoscopically, but the long-term results suggest lower cure rates and higher urinary tract complications when compared to the open methods. At present an MRC trial is underway to clarify this. Marshall-Marchetti and Krantz described the original colposuspension. The sutures were inserted into the periosteum of the superior ramus of pubis, and although the subjective cure rates are similar there was a high incidence of osteitis pubis, hence this procedure for primary or secondary GSI is not very popular these days.

Suburethral sling procedures are indicated in severe recurrent GSI and intrinsic urethral failure. The slings (pigskin, meshes, autologous grafts) have all been described. The principle is to pass the strip of material underneath the urethra or bladder neck and anchor it to the anterior abdominal wall. The success rates are difficult to assess because of previous surgery, but are reported to be about 80% in the short term. The main complications are higher rates of DI (30%), voiding difficulties and graft erosion (with the synthetic material).

A newer method called tension-free vaginal tape (TVT) has gained popularity in recent years. This is different in that the sling is a tape placed at the level of the mid-urethra. This comes from the idea that GSI results from failure of the pubo-urethral ligaments in the mid-urethra. The advantage of the tape is that it is self-retaining and can be inserted under local or regional anaesthesia. It is successful in more than 80% of cases, but there seems to be a high bladder trauma rate (8%) and a study is currently underway to compare it to colposuspension.

Anterior colporrhaphy with Kelly or Pacey buttressing sutures is successful in 40–70% cases. It should only be performed in the presence of significant uterovaginal prolapse, not as a first line procedure for GSI. The first operation performed should be the one that offers the best chance of a long-term cure. The operation is performed by making an inverted V-shaped or diamond incision along the anterior vaginal wall to expose the vesicovaginal space. Once the space is exposed, the vaginal fascia is separated from the vesical fascia by blunt and sharp dissection. The redundant vaginal skin is removed. The interrupted buttress sutures are then inserted either side of the bladder into the pubocervical and vesical fascia with vicryl to create a firm buttress. The vagina is then closed with a continuous suture of vicryl.

Stamey's needle bladder neck suspension or a modification may be useful in the surgically difficult patient. However the long-term results are poor.

Periurethral bulk-enhancing agents, such as glutaraldehyde cross-linked bovine (GAX) collagen, macroplastic or autologous fat may be indicated in surgically difficult or medically unfit patients. They may also have a role in women undergoing repeat procedures or with intrinsic sphincter deficiency. The bulking agents increase the urethral closure pressure and achieve better apposition of the urethral epithelium. Complications are uncommon (urinary infections occurring in about 20%), but repeat procedures may be necessary. Long-term continence rates are still not well defined, but cure rates of 40–60% have been reported. The injections are made either transurethrally or peri-urethrally under cystoscopic guidance.

Complex surgical procedures, like artificial sphincter, neourethra or urinary diversion may be the ultimate option in intractable recurrent sphincter incompetence.

Further reading

Slade R *et al.* (1998) Urinary incontinence. *Key Topics in Obstetrics and Gynaecology*, pp. 135–141. BIOS Scientific Publishers Ltd, Oxford.

Bidmead J, Cardozo L (1998) Detrusor instability. RCOG Pace Review No. 98/03. Royal College of Obstetricians and Gynaecologists, London.

Bidmead J, Cardozo L (2000) Surgery for genuine stress incontinence. In: Studd J (ed.), *Progress in Obstetrics and Gynaecology*, Vol. 14, pp. 329–358. Churchill Livingstone, Edinburgh.

Cardozo L (1995) Urinary incontinence and other disorders of the lower urinary tract in women. In: Whitfield CR (ed.), *Dewhurst's Textbook of Obstetrics and Gynaecology for Postgraduates*, 5th edn, pp. 653–680. Blackwell Scientific Publications, Oxford.

Cardozo L, Hill S (1996) Urinary incontinence. RCOG Pace Review No. 96/09. Royal College of Obstetricians and Gynaecologists, London.

Jarvis JG (2000) Treatment of detrusor instability and urge incontinence. In: Studd J (ed.), *Progress in Obstetrics and Gynaecology*, Vol. 14, pp. 359–371. Churchill Livingstone, Edinburgh.

Ulmsten U, Johnson P, Rezapour M (1999) A three-year follow up of tension free vaginal tape for surgical treatment of female stress urinary incontinence. *Br. J. Obstet. Gynaecol.* **106**: 345–350.

CIRCUIT 3

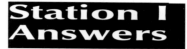

Answer I1

It looks like a diamniotic-monochorionic pregnancy. Though the dividing membrane is visible, it is difficult to comment on the chorionicity. As only one placenta is visible, it is more likely to be monochorionic. In diamniotic-monochorionic twins, the dividing membranes form the 'T-sign', while in diamniotic-dichorionic twins they form the 'lambda-sign'.

It is important to determine the chorionicity because monochorionic twins have more complications compared to dichorionic twins. If there was discordant growth, the knowledge of chorionicity may help to distinguish between an IUGR baby and twin-to-twin transfusion syndrome. Similarly, if a congenital anomaly were noted in one twin it would help to predict the likely outcome if a selective termination was required.

Answer I2

I would begin by explaining the scan findings of a twin pregnancy that agrees with her dates and makes her 13 weeks pregnant. The twins look to be in separate sacs, but they appear to be sharing the same placenta. Both the heartbeats have been identified and although there is only a minimal chance of one of them miscarrying, the risk is five-times greater in monozygous twins.

I would need to provide her with a lot of information about multiple pregnancy and its potential complications, management and the delivery. I would also need to discuss her desire for a home birth and strongly discourage it.

With regard to the pregnancy, I would begin by explaining that she was more likely to suffer with the unpleasant symptoms of pregnancy such as nausea, tiredness, heartburn, backache, haemorrhoids and varicose veins. If her heartburn were resistant to simple antacids I would recommend commencing her on a H_2 blocker such as ranitidine. This appears to be safe, and although it crosses the placenta, does not appear to be teratogenic. It is also highly effective with few maternal side effects. Obviously, I would also advise her about avoiding spicy foods, alcohol and smoking and talk about her posture and position in bed. She is also more likely to become anaemic, and although iron supplementation is often recommended as it restores normal values, there is no evidence to say iron supplementation is actually beneficial to mother or baby.

I would then need to discuss screening with her. She is 40 years old, and her risks of having a Down's syndrome baby are approximately 1 in 55 (1 in 110 for a singleton pregnancy). In view of the fact that this is a twin pregnancy I would not recommend the use of a triple test as a risk estimate for Down's syndrome, because it has a poor detection rate. She is 13 weeks so it could be possible to look at the nuchal translucency for a risk estimate. This appears to be as effective in detecting Down's syndrome as in singleton pregnancies, but has a higher false positive rate. If she wished for a definitive diagnosis she would need an amniocentesis in a tertiary referral centre. This is because it may be difficult to determine which is the affected baby if the results were abnormal, and if an abnormal baby was detected and they share the same placenta, selective termination would be extremely hazardous. Another consideration is the increased risk of miscarriage compared to singleton pregnancy following an amniocentesis. I would, however, recommend a detailed scan at 20 weeks because of the increased risks of neural tube defects, cardiac abnormalities and bowel atresias with twins.

With regard to her antenatal care, I would recommend that this be shared care rather than community led because the risks of complication are twice as great in twin pregnancy. After her 20-week scan I would advise growth scans every 2 weeks to look for poor growth in one fetus, or discordant growth that may be an indicator of twin-to-twin transfusion syndrome.

I would explain that she is more at risk of premature labour (five times), but this is often difficult to predict. I would not recommend routine vaginal examinations or scans because they have not been shown to be of benefit. Similarly, there is no evidence to suggest that prophylactic betamimetic agents or bed rest are of use. In fact, bed rest may be detrimental. There is no evidence to suggest that prophylactic corticosteroids are useful, their effects may be limited.

I would also explain that she is at much higher risk of pregnancy-induced hypertension, gestational diabetes, polyhydramnios, placenta praevia and post partum haemorrhage. My advice to see her every 2 weeks would also allow measurement of her blood pressure and urinalysis to look for the development of these complications.

Specifically, with monochorionic twins there are increased risks of fetal malformations, intrauterine growth restriction (IUGR), twin-to-twin transfusion syndrome, fetal acardia, cord entanglement, and a higher perinatal mortality rate (2.5 times greater). There is also the possibility of conjoined twins in monoamniotic-monochorionic twins.

With regard to her labour, at this point I would not discuss it in great detail except that I would recommend delivery in a hospital environment and certainly would not sanction her desire for a home birth because of the risks stated above.

Answer 13

The likely diagnosis is twin–twin transfusion syndrome (fetofetal transfusion syndrome); this complicates 10–15% of monochorionic twin pregnancies.

In monochorionic placentation, vascular anastomoses connecting the circulations of the two twins are usually present. These can be vein to vein, artery to artery and artery to vein. Arteriovenous vascular connections cause twin–twin transfusion syndrome. It leads to anaemia, growth restriction and extreme oligohydramnios in the 'donor' twin, and polycythaemia and severe polyhydramnios in the 'recipient'. It usually presents with severe polyhydramnios during the second trimester. The fetal loss rate is very high (>80%) mainly due to extremely preterm labour. There is also significant perinatal morbidity from acquired brain injury in utero and the complications of pre-term delivery.

Although it is suspected by the scan appearances, it can only be diagnosed by finding an inter-twin difference in haemoglobin concentration of greater than 5 g/dl, and a birthweight difference of greater than 20%. However, the common cause for these differences is discordant growth restriction in dichorionic twins, chronic hypoxaemia inducing polycythaemia in the growth-restricted fetus. Before confirming the diagnosis of twin–twin transfusion, it is important to inspect the placenta and to ensure that the smaller twin has the lower haemoglobin.

During the antenatal period, it may be suspected by the acute onset of severe polyhydramnios and discordant size of the fetuses. Ultrasound using colour flow and Doppler studies may be useful showing similar umbilical artery waveforms in both fetuses. Colour Doppler can also demonstrate vascular anastomoses, which with other clinical and ultrasound features are useful to diagnose it during the antenatal period. Arterio-arterial anastomoses seem to protect against its development.

Once the diagnosis is suspected, referral to a tertiary unit is advisable. The usual management is to perform serial therapeutic amniocentesis to reduce the amniotic fluid volume in the polyhydramniotic sac. Indomethacin has been used to reduce polyhydramnios and to prolong the pregnancy, but its main drawback is the effect on the fetus and neonate following prolonged use. Laser coagulation of the anastomotic vessels in the placenta and septostomy have also been performed with limited success.

Answer 14

This is a rare dysmorphic problem unique to monochorionic twins with vascular anastomoses. There may be some development of the head and thorax with well formed limbs or the fetus may present as an amorphous mass without much resemblance to a human fetus. The acardiac fetus depends on the blood supply from its co-twin, which requires both artery–artery and vein–vein anastomoses in the placenta. Poorly oxygenated arterial blood from the co-twin passes in a pulsatile and retrograde direction through the umbilical artery to the acardiac twin (twin reversed arterial perfusion, TRAP).

Answer 15

I will check the chorionicity of the twin pregnancy first. Then I will tell her that she is carrying two babies. In about 50% of cases of twin pregnancies diagnosed in the first trimester, one of the fetuses is lost, and in the majority of cases the other continues to grow. This 'vanishing twin' presents with first trimester bleeding in 25% of cases, but remains asymptomatic in the rest (75%). When one fetus is lost in the first trimester, resorption occurs. If it happens in the second trimester, the remains of the baby become paper-like and flattened (*fetus papyraceous*) by pressure from the membranes of the surviving fetus. This presents a problem in that the *fetus papyraceous* has to be registered as a stillbirth.

Answer 16

In this circumstance there are possible risks to both the surviving fetus and the mother. The surviving fetus would be at risk of intrauterine growth restriction and even death prenatally. When one twin dies there is a 25% risk of necrotic neurological and renal lesions with a similar risk of death to the other twin. Other fetal risks include cerebral palsy, microcephaly, multicystic encephalopathy, renal cortical necrosis and aplasia cutis after birth (the possible explanation is infarction of various organs due to haemodynamic imbalance or passage of emboli of thromboplastic substances from the dead twin via placental anastomoses). The main concern for the mother, apart from the psychological morbidity is the development of disseminated intravascular coagulation (DIC). Thankfully, this is rare, and DIC usually does not occur before 5 weeks.

The management includes frequent surveillance of the surviving twin (ultrasound scans, biophysical profile etc.) and weekly measurement of maternal coagulation profiles. Steroids can be administered if delivery is considered, but this should only be done if there is an appropriate obstetric indication. Early delivery does not improve perinatal outcome. Fetal blood sampling may be necessary to identify anaemia and to allow for a rescue transfusion. Vaginal delivery is preferable. Neonatal cranial ultrasound is recommended after delivery.

Further reading

Enkin M, Keirse MJNC, Neilson J et al. (2000) A guide to effective care in pregnancy and childbirth, 3rd edn, pp. 95–107 and 141–147. Oxford University Press, Oxford.

Neilson JP (1995) Multiple pregnancy. In: Whitfield CR (ed.), *Dewhurst's Textbook of Obstetrics and Gynaecology for Postgraduates*, 5th edn, pp. 439–453. Blackwell Science, Oxford.

Slade R et al. (1998) Multiple Pregnancy. *Key Topics in Obstetrics and Gynaecology*, pp. 248–250. BIOS Scientific Publishers Ltd, Oxford.

Taylor MJO, Fisk NM (2000) Multiple pregnancy. *The Obstetrician and Gynaecologist* 2(4): 4–10.

CIRCUIT 3

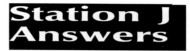
Answer J1

The basic principle behind the use of diathermy is the generation of heat using electricity.

When an electric current passes from a large diameter conductor to a small diameter conductor it experiences resistance (impedance). The result of this is the generation of heat, because at this point the current density is higher. A similar thing happens when an electric current meets with resistance from other causes such as body tissues. When in contact with tissues, a metal conductor (active electrode) will generate heat. The smaller the point of contacts of the conductor with the tissue the greater the current density and effect generated.

When introducing electricity into the body we need to ensure that there is a way for the electricity to return to earth. This necessitates using a pad (normally strapped to the thigh in gynaecology) with a large surface area, providing a low current density, which should not therefore generate heat. If this were to partially come off to create a smaller surface area, then a burn would result at the site of the return plate.

The current used is not directly mains electricity as this may result in fibrillation of the heart (up to 100 Hz). Hence, the mains electricity is passed to a generator which produces safer high frequency waveforms (500 000 Hz).

The way that the current is generated depends on the end results desired. If the waveform is a constant sinusoidal pattern it will produce a cutting current. The result of a cutting current, delivered through a fine point is that the high current density generated causes the surrounding tissues to explode with little thermal spread (the tissues are vapourized quickly and this removes the excess heat to reduce lateral thermal damage). To generate a coagulation effect the waveform is intermittent and pulsed. This provides the tissues with some time to cool off between energy bursts.

These principles relate to monopolar diathermy. With bipolar diathermy, instead of relying on a return plate to complete the electric circuit, this is done within the bipolar forceps. The current passes down one side of the forceps through the tissue and then returns to the generator through the other side of the forceps. This allows highly precise coagulation at low power settings, without thermal spread and damage to other tissues.

Safety is a very important issue. The return electrode plate should be placed on the patient as near to the surgical site as possible. Ideally it should not be sited over a scar or the site of a metal implant. The plate should be large and totally in contact with the skin, preferably over tissues with a good blood supply. Sites should be avoided with excessive hair, dry skin or irregular body contours. The pad should not be entirely dry, because if it is and it gets into contact with any fluids, the fluid will provide better conductivity and a burn may result. Most modern pads are disposable and come with a self-adhesive conductive gel already applied. Once the pads have been applied it is essential that they do not get wet with skin preparation. Some generators can monitor the return pads and if they detect a problem the current will not be produced.

In laparoscopic surgery it is essential that the metal instruments are insulated to the tips to prevent current leakage where it is not desired. They should always be inspected prior to use and the insulation sleeves checked. When using diathermy at laparoscopy the points of the instruments should always be in view to ensure that there is no touching of other instruments (direct coupling) that could conduct the current elsewhere. Diathermy should only be activated when in contact with tissues. Metal and plastic cannulas and fixation screws should not be mixed because this can generate capacitive coupling. The lowest power settings should be used.

Answer J2

A suture is a thread that either approximates and maintains tissues until the natural healing process has provided a sufficient level of wound strength, or compresses blood vessels in order to stop bleeding. They are probably the largest group of devices implanted in humans.

Sutures are of different types and sizes, and made in different ways.

Sutures can be divided into two groups, non-absorbable and absorbable. Non-absorbable sutures are not dissolved or decomposed by the body's natural actions. Such sutures are generally not naturally occurring materials (except silk); some (silk and nylon) while being classified as non-absorbable actually dissolve after very long periods of time. On the other hand, absorbable sutures are temporary due to their ability to be "absorbed" or decomposed by the natural reaction of the body to foreign substances. Not all absorbable sutures have the same resistance level to absorption, but each can be designed or treated to obtain the desired decomposition rate.

Suture sizes are represented by a number that equals the diameter of the suture. The numbers range (in descending order) from 10 to 1 and then 1–0 to 12–0, 10 is the thickest and 12–0 the thinnest (its diameter is smaller than a human hair). The metric number represents the diameter of the stitch in tenths of a millimetre, the smaller the size, the less tensile strength the material has.

Another factor to be taken into account is the effect of inserting the suture into the tissue. If the suture is of a rough type (e.g. braided), the tissue will swell more and is more susceptible to infection than if a smooth suture (e.g. monofilament) is used.

With regard to the sutures illustrated:

Dexon
This is 2.0 (3 metric) Dexon, which is braided Polyglycolic acid with a Polycaprolate coating system. It is mounted on a half circle needle, 40 mm long with a taper cut point. The stitch is 2 colours and it is 75 cm long. Dexon is an absorbable suture. The needle-point is taper cut which is a combination of a cutting and round-bodied needle. It is useful where tissue penetration is required, and is a multipurpose heavy needle. It is braided to ensure excellent handling and knotting. Dexon is degraded slightly quicker than Vicryl, overall approximately 60% remains up to 21–28 days and the material is not totally absorbed from the wound until 60–90 days.

Mersilk
This is 2.0 (3 metric) braided Silk, on a 55 mm straight needle with a cutting point. The stitch is black in colour and it is 1 m long, 55 mm is the shortest straight needle available. This is a non-absorbable stitch. Cutting needles are useful wherever tough or dense tissue needs to be sutured.

PDS II
This is 1 (4 metric) PDS, which is Polydioxanone. It is mounted on a half circle needle, 30 mm long with a round-bodied tip. The colour of the stitch is violet and it is 70 cm long. PDS is a monofilament absorbable suture. It is slowly absorbed by hydrolysis with minimal tissue reaction. It holds its strength twice as long as coated Vicryl and is stronger than other monofilaments. It loses its strength in 50–60 days and is only completely absorbed in 6 months (180 days). The smooth monofilament is designed to minimize tissue resistance during suture placement.

Monocryl
This is 2.0 (3 metric) Monocryl, which is Poliglecaprone 25. It is mounted on a half circle needle, 30 mm long with a round-bodied tip. The stitch is violet in colour and it is 70 cm long. This is a monofilament absorbable suture. Round-bodied needles are not designed to cut tissues, rather split them. They are useful in soft tissues.

Chromic catgut
This is 1 (5 metric) chromic catgut. It is mounted on a half circle needle, 30 mm long with a round bodied tip and it is 75 cm long. Catgut is an absorbable suture manufactured from the submucosal layer of sheep intestine or the serosal layer of beef intestine. It is sterilized by gamma irradiation. It loses half of its tensile strength within 2 weeks (11–14 days), and all its strength in 4 weeks. Absorption may take up to 90 days to complete and it can generate marked tissue reaction, but less than plain catgut. It is the thickest stitch of all those illustrated. It is being replaced by synthetic materials.

Ethilon
This is 2.0 (3 metric) Ethilon, which is Polyamide 6 Monofilament. It is mounted on a straight needle, 55 mm long with a cutting point. The stitch is blue in colour and it is 55 cm long. It is a non-absorbable monofilament suture. It may be used for wound closure either as interrupted or a sub-cuticular stitch.

Prolene

This is 0 (3.5 metric) Polypropylene monofilament. It is mounted on a 30 mm long J needle with a heavy tapercut point. Tapercut points combine the initial penetration of a cutting needle with the minimized trauma of a round bodied needle. The cutting tip is limited to the point of the needle, which then tapers out to merge smoothly with the round shaft. The stitch is blue in colour and it is 1 m long. Like Ethilon, it is a non-absorbable monofilament suture. It is unaffected by tissue enzymes and ideal for use in infected areas.

Vicryl Rapide

This is 2.0 (3 metric) Polyglactin braided absorbable suture. It is mounted on a 35 mm long half circle needle with a tapercut point. The stitch is white (undyed) and it is 1.2 m long. It is an absorbable suture. It is braided to ensure excellent handling and knotting. It has the same properties as Vicryl but due to the sterilization process, using gamma irradiation, the tensile strength is reduced between 10 and 14 days and it is therefore fully absorbed by 35–42 days.

Answer J3

1. This is a hysteroscope. It looks like a small diameter one (2–4 mm) that might be useful for outpatient hysteroscopy. It can be used to investigate things such as menorrhagia in women over 45, post menopausal bleeding following abnormal transvaginal scans, or be used to ensure correct dilatation and a normal cavity prior to any of the third generation endometrial ablative techniques. The sleeve with it is an operating sheath. The two-way taps allow fluid to enter through one side and be sucked away through the other. The other channel allows instruments such as small scissors or biopsy forceps to be introduced.

2. This is a 10 mm laparoscope. It can be used for diagnostic purposes such as for investigating pelvic pain, ectopic pregnancies, to assess tubal patency and for overseeing laparoscopic operations. It is the largest diameter laparoscope available and provides better definition than the smaller laparoscopes.

   The other instrument with it is a Veress needle. This is inserted, normally through the umbilicus and is attached to the carbon dioxide insufflator. It creates the pneumoperitoneum that subsequently allows the laparoscopic procedure to be performed.

Appendix A

Biochemical reference intervals ('normal values' and therapeutic ranges)

Substance	Sample	Reference interval
Acid phosphate (total)	S	1–5 IU/l
Acid phosphatase (prostatic)	S	0–1 IU/l
Adrenocorticotrophin (ACTH)	P	<10–80 ng/l
Alanine-amino transferase (ALT)	P	5–35 IU/l
Albumin	P	35–50 g/l
Aldosterone	P	100-500 pmol/l
Alkaline phosphatase	P	30–300 IU/l
α-amylase	P	0–180 somogyi units/dl
Angiotensin II	P	5–35 pmol/l
Antidiuretic hormone (ADH)	P	0.9–4.6 pmol/l
Aspartate-amino transferase (AST)	P	5–35 IU/l
Bicarbonate	P	24–30 mmol/l
Bilirubin	P	3–17 µmol/l
Calcitonin	P	<27 pmol/l
Calcium (ionized)	P	1.0–1.25 mmol/l
Calcium (total)	P	2.12–2.65 mmol/l
Chloride	P	95–105 mmol/l
Cholesterol	P	3.9–7.8 mmol/l
Cortisol	P	a.m. 280–700 nmol/l
		p.m. 140–280 nmol/l
Creatine kinase (CPK)	P	M25–195 IU/l
		F25–170 IU/l
Creatinine	P	70–150 µmol/l
5'-nucleotidase (5 NT)	P	3–17 IU/l
Folate	S	5–63 nmol/l (2.1–2.8 µg/l)
Follicle-stimulating hormone (FSH)	P/S	2–8 U/l
Gamma-glutamyl trans-peptidase		M11–51 IU/l
(γ-GT)	P	F 7–33 IU/l
Glucose (fasting)	P	4–6 mmol/l
Growth hormone	P	<20 mU/l
Iron	S	M 14–31 µmol/l
		F 11–30 µmol/l
Lactate dehydrogenase (LDH)	P	240–525 IU/l
Luteinizing hormone (LH)		
(pre-menopausal)	P	6–13 U/l
Magnesium	P	0.75–1.05 mmol/l
Osmolality	P	278–305 mosm/kg
Parathormone	P	<0.1–0.73 µg/l
Phosphate (inorganic)	P	0.8–1.45 mmol/l